The Origin and Onset of Thrombus Disease

Collapsed balancing function of immune cells and triggering factors

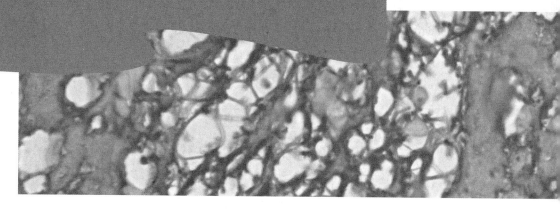

LeMin Wang

人民卫生出版社
PMPH PEOPLE'S MEDICAL PUBLISHING HOUSE

图书在版编目（CIP）数据

血栓病的起源与发生：免疫细胞平衡功能崩溃与启动机制
=The Origin and Onset of Thrombus Disease：collapsed balancing
function of immune cells and triggering factors：英文 / 王乐民著．
—北京：人民卫生出版社，2017
ISBN 978-7-117-25335-2

Ⅰ.①血…　Ⅱ.①王…　Ⅲ.①血栓栓塞 - 研究 - 英文
Ⅳ.①R543

中国版本图书馆 CIP 数据核字（2017）第 258210 号

| 人卫智网 | www.ipmph.com | 医学教育、学术、考试、健康，购书智慧智能综合服务平台 |
| 人卫官网 | www.pmph.com | 人卫官方资讯发布平台 |

The Origin and Onset of Thrombus Disease

Collapsed balancing function of immune cells and triggering factors

著　　者：王乐民
出版发行：人民卫生出版社（中继线 010-59780011）
地　　址：北京市朝阳区潘家园南里 19 号
邮　　编：100021
E - mail：pmph @ pmph.com
购书热线：010-59787592　010-59787584　010-65264830
印　　刷：北京盛通印刷股份有限公司
经　　销：新华书店
开　　本：787×1092　1/16　印张：15
字　　数：365 千字
版　　次：2017 年 11 月第 1 版　2017 年 11 月第 1 版第 1 次印刷
标准书号：ISBN 978-7-117-25335-2/R · 25336
定　　价：180.00 元

打击盗版举报电话：010-59787491　E-mail：WQ @ pmph.com
（凡属印装质量问题请与本社市场营销中心联系退换）

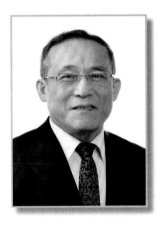

LeMin Wang, MD, PhD
Professor of Department of Cardiology
Tongji Hospital of Tongji University
Shanghai, China

Treatises as the editor

1. Acute pulmonary embolism. Helongjiang: Helongjiang science and technology publishing house, 1999.
2. Pathophysiology of cardiovascular disease(Tranlsation). Helongjiang: Helongjiang science and technology publishing house, 2000.
3. Pulmonary embolism and deep venous thrombosis. Beijing: People's Medical Publishing House, 2001.
4. Coronary heart disease. Beijing:People's Medical Publishing House, 2003.
5. Pulmonary circulation diseases. Beijing: People's Medical Publishing House, 2007.
6. Pulmonary embolism and deep venous thrombosis. second edition. Beijing: People's Medical Publishing House, 2008.

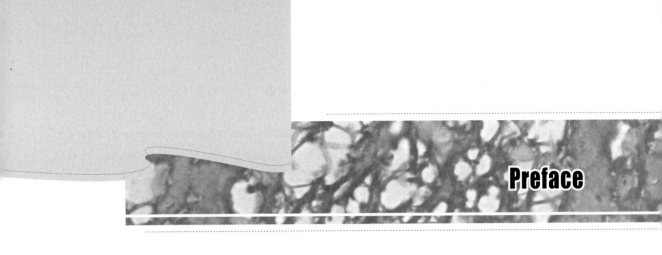

Preface

The aim of this book is to summarize research data, which support a central role of alterations in immune functions in thrombosis development. Whilst venous (red) and arterial (white) thrombi differ histologically, their upstream initiating factors are similar. Venous thrombi, whether familial or acquired, result from a defensive mechanism to prevent the passage of intravenous microorganisms or malignant cells by the formation of biological filters. Such filters then also trap red blood cells, hence resulting in typical venous red thrombosis. Arterial thrombosis results from endothelial damage leading to platelet adhesion. The rupture of the atherosclerosis soft plaque cap and superficial anabrotic damage to the endothelium may result from the effects of reactive oxygen species or cytokines released from neutrophils activated in response to the microorganisms that have entered the bloodstream following the collapse of the immune cell balance function. Thus venous thrombosis results from activation of the body's new defensive mechanism, whilst arterial thrombosis results from a failure of defensive mechanism to clear pathogens.

This book brings together extensive studies of the author conducted over the past couple of decades into the origins and pathogenesis of thrombosis with publications in a range of leading international journals. We have conducted studies in a variety of clinical groups and on different experimental models, using a range of technical approaches including genomics, proteomics, immunology, microbiology and cytology. We also analyzed internal and external causes of acquired and familiar venous thrombosis and proposed origin and onset of venous thrombus diseases and its triggering factors. Based on genomics and immunocytological research findings, we proposed collapsed immune cell balance function as the origin of arterial thrombus diseases and concluded that exogenous microorganisms may be the triggering factor of arterial thrombosis.

The recognition of natural phenomena originates from curiosity and observation, gradually from shallower to the deeper and from the surface to the center, rising spirally. It is the same with recognizing diseases. However, it is the development of the times that provides the possibility to understand the micro structures and functions of diseases. "The origin and onset of thrombus Diseases" welcomes any comments, suggestions or criticisms from readers with common interest in research or clinical areas.

This book is dedicated to all graduate students of our thrombosis research team. Their multi-dimensional perspective work verifies the origin and onset of thromboembolic disease and its immune mechanism. The team members includes: Dr. Fan Yang, Dr. Qianglin Duan, Dr. Wei Lv, Dr. Zhu Gong, Dr. Haoming Song, Dr. Lin Zhou, Dr. Yanli Song, Dr. Wenwen Yan, Dr. Hao Wang, Dr. Qiang Wang, Dr. Guiyuan Li, Dr. Yun Jin, Dr. Siwan Wen, Dr. Zhiru Ge, Dr. Kebin Cheng, Dr.Mei Fu, Dr. Xiaoyu Zhang, Dr. Chunyu Huang, Dr. Yuan Xie, Dr.Jinghua Tan, Dr. Qi Yu, Dr. Yixin Chen, Dr. Chuanrong Li.

Acknowledgment

I greatly appreciate Profs. Jinfa Jiang, Wenju Xu, Xianghua Yi, Haiying Wan from Tongji Hospital of Tongji University for data collection and detection. I also give thanks to Prof. Yu Zhang from electron microscopy center of Fudan Univserity, Profs. Hengjun Gao and Xiaoying Shen from South Gene Chip Center for their platform. Profs. Huikang Zhao and Jing Chen made great effort in image production. Guanghe Li helped to edit the draft. Many thanks should also be given to my parents, my wife and friends. Finally, I specially appreciate Dr. Qianglin Duan, Prof. Shulin Liu and Prof. Anthony Dart .Monash University, Australia.for their kind help in English usage.

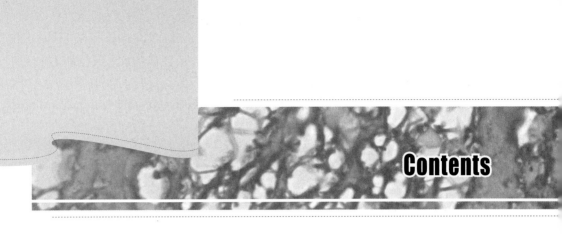

Contents

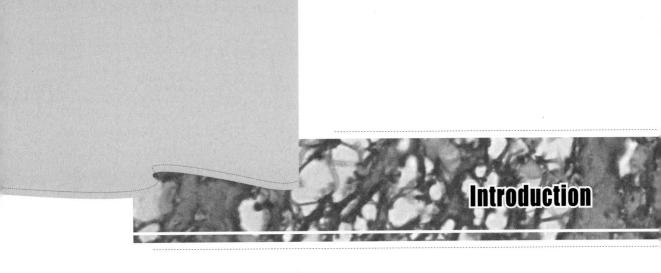

Introduction

Thrombosis, in arterial or venous vessels, is a common disease with a high morbidity worldwide. Since all the organs and tissues are supported by the blood circulation system, thrombus can occur in any part of the body and is related to a diverse range of clinical disciplines. Additionally, the presence of arterial or venous thrombosis is indicative of a subversive imbalance in the body defense system.

In 1856, the German pathologist Rudolf Virchow first identified 3 main factors responsible for thrombosis, subsequently known as Virchow's triad, including hypercoagulability of the blood, damage of the vessel wall and hemodynamic alterations such as stasis. Virchow's triad remains the paradigm guiding clinical practice today. For decades, there have been many international guidelines on the prevention, clinic diagnosis and treatment of arterial and venous thrombi, proposing risk factors and risk stratification of arterial or venous thrombus. Thrombosis in the coronary, cerebral, peripheral arteries and pulmonary arteries and in deep vein still remains at a high incidence worldwide, so different interventions and prevention measures have been adopted. Patients with thrombotic diseases may suffer from the sequelae and young patients often die from thrombosis.

The advantages of the refinement of the clinical branches for the convenience of intensive work are self-evident. However, for the specifics of the refinement, the viewpoints of the practitioners are limited: they tend to focus on the divided parts, so the human body integrality is often cut into pieces. As a result, the knowledge is often fragmentary and the internal integrity of science is split, largely owing to the limitation of recognition about the disease, which, whether in the arterial or venous system, is usually a local expression of a systemic disease instead of abnormities in one particular organ or a single vessel branch. Therefore, it should be analyzed in a holistic view rather than at the specific thrombotic organ or location to search for the leakage.

For the evidence-based medicine of thrombotic diseases, risk factors could be evaluated based on the observed clinical manifestations. However, they are not the essence of the genesis of the disease and so may not reveal the causality of the disease. Statistical data may suggest the causality but may not be correct. In order to comprehend the thrombosis correctly, the underlying mechanisms should be explored.

Much about thrombosis is still a mystery, such as its origins. A full picture of the thrombosis should be obtained with a holographic thinking instead of the linear or planar thinking. Meanwhile, the mechanisms behind the development of the thrombotic disease should be revealed, and the processes of pathogenesis from the clinical manifestation to the nature of the disease should be explored. There are needs of evidence, epitomization of medical knowledge, integration of multiple disciplines, as well as vertical and horizontal fusions. Not only a deep understanding of the clinical practices should be established to raise query in clinics, but also the advanced methods in modern medicine should be adopted to deal with the massive data acquired. In the meanwhile, rational thinking and hierarchical analysis on a philosophical level are indispensable, which is just like exploring the unknown mysteries of the universe.

Venous thrombosis is triggered by infected cells or malignant cells, while arterial thrombosis may be triggered by pathogenic microorganisms. However, the underlying condition of both venous and arterial thrombosis is the same. Both thrombosis occur under the collapse of the immune cell balance function, which is the common kernel of the origin of thrombus disease. The venous thrombosis results from the substitution of own new defense morphology, but the arterial thrombosis results from the self repair of the injured endarterium. The different expressing ways both follow common law of biology, which benefits self stabilization and continuity of living bodies. However, the local beneficial defense and repair lead eventually to harmful thrombotic clogging, and the activation of blood coagulation factors only makes the defense and repair firmer.

The immune system, consisting of a variety of organs, tissues, cells and their products, which is to timely and effectively remove deleterious factors from the body. Collapsed immune cell balance function refers to non-function or significant dysfunction of immune cells. There are short-term inhibition of immune cell function and long-term significant dysfunction of immune cell function. Systemic immnune cell balance function collapse inevitably results in subversive disease, including thrombotic diseases. Even in the presence of thrombus risk factors, thrombosis will not occur in an individual with a healthy immune cell balance function.

The nervous, endocrine and immune systems paly important roles in regulating internal physiological activities and self equilibrium as a whole. The neuro-endocrine-immune regulation is a huge development of the macro-control theory of modern medicine. The innate and adaptive immune functions are both under the mediation of the vegetative nerve and endocrine systems. Thus, immune cell balancing function collapse is associated with the state of over stress, in which transmitters secreted by excessively activated sympathetic nerves can decrease the number of lymphocytes, inhibit the receptors of lymphocytes, increase the number of phagocytes, and activate the receptors of phagocytes. This phenomenon is obvious in middle-aged patients with thrombotic diseases. The immune function can be influenced by many factors such as advanced age, infection, temperature, barometric pressure, drugs as well as food balance, with which thrombotic diseases in elder people are often related. It should be extended to the upstream of the disease from the middle and lower reaches to prevent the thrombotic disease, to decrease the incidence and to increase the cure rate. Hence, it is needed to lower the stress level inside human body and restore the balance of neuroendocrine functions, which is the new content of prevention, treatment and rehabilitation of thrombotic diseases.

Part I
Venous thrombus

Chapter 1

The origin and onset of acute venous thrombus

Immune cell balancing function collapse refers to no function or significant dysfunction of immune cells, involving mostly T lymphocytes. Under the condition of immune cell balancing function collapse, acute venous thrombosis originates from intravenous immune adhesive inflammatory reactions triggered by infected cells/malignant tumor cells, which happens throughout the whole process of genesis of venous thrombosis.

Thrombotic inflammation, including infectious inflammation (by pathogenic microorganism) and non-infectious inflammation (by malignant tumor cells), is a defensive response. The outcome of inflammation depends on the strength of immune cell balancing function. With the condition of immune cell balancing function collapse, the human body loses the function of eliminating intravenous infected cells/ malignant tumor cells timely and effectively. Thus, integrin subunits β1, β2 and β3 on the membrane of platelets and white blood cells are activated to combine with the ligand fibrinogen into a reversible mesh-like structure, which is like the intravenous biological filter and acts as physical defense of the human body to prevent the infected cells/malignant tumor cells in the distal veins from flowing back. During the process of defense, blood cells, mainly red blood cells, stagnate and fulfill the filter, which stops the blood flow in the local veins and thus results in venous thrombotic diseases.

The process, in which integrin β2 and β3 receptors on white blood cells or platelets membrane combine with their ligands fibrinogen, is reversible and easy to be disintegrated. Thus, only under the condition of stasis can the biological filter form. Otherwise, the combinations will be impacted into pieces by the quick blood flow. Integrin β2 on the membrane of neutrophils combines with its ligand Factor X to Factor Xa, activates coagulation factors and converts fibrinogen in the filamentous sieve into fibrin, which makes the intravenous biological filter firm. Fibrinoid inflammation is the pathological manifestation of venous thrombosis.

In people with a sound immune function, infected cells/malignant tumor cells can be removed timely and effectively, which makes it unnecessary to start the intravenous biological filter to act as a compensatory physical defense. Thus, acute venous thrombotic events will not take place under such circumstances. Patients with collapsed immune cell balancing functions are a group of people,who have particularly high risks of venous thrombosis. Meanwhile, anyone who has venous thromboembolism may have infected cells/malignant tumor cells in veins, which may trigger the genesis of venous thrombosis. Only under the condition of immune cell balancing function collapse, the risk factors, such as advanced age, infection, trauma, surgery, autoimmune disease, long-time bedding, pregnancy, delivery as well as long trip syndrome, may cause venous thrombosis. However, even with definable risk factors, venous thromboembolism usually does not form in people with sound immune functions.

(Published: Int J Clin Exp Med 2015;8(11):19804-19814)

Chapter 2

The answer to the onset of acute venous thrombus

1. Questions from clinics

Venous thromboembolism (VTE) includes pulmonary thromboembolism (PE) and deep venous thrombosis (DVT). Venous thromboembolisms that could be diagnosed in clinics are called dominant VTE. The clinical spectrum of VTE is relatively wide, because VTE can occur in different organs and tissues. However, dormant VTE that is hard to be diagnosed in clinics is often found in autopsy. VTE, including cerebral cortical vein, cerebral venous sinus thrombosis, acute PE, chronic thromboembolic pulmonary hypertension (CTEPH), hepatic venular occlusive disease, Butchart's syndrome, mesenteric venous thrombosis, pelvic venous thrombosis, DVT and PE after surgeries as well as clinically common lower limb DVTs, distributes in diverse clinical disciplines and is a disease faced by almost all the clinical disciplines. Among them, PE has become a global medical care problem due to its high morbidity, misdiagnosis rate and mortality [1, 2]. VTE can be divided into two categories, genetic VTE and acquired VTE. According to the results of epidemiological investigations, the incidence of genetic VTE is relatively low, while most of the VTEs are acquired VTEs. Both of them can be called symptomatic VTE (Figure 2-1-1,2,3) and are hard to be distinguished.

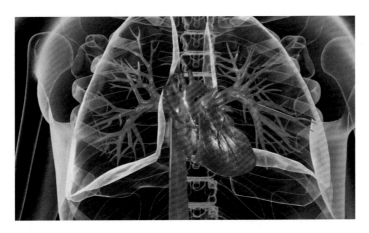

Figure 2-1-1   Simulation diagram of pulmonary thromboembolism

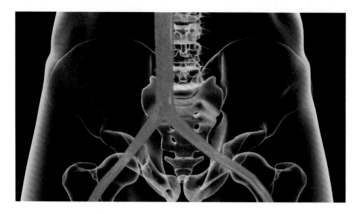

Figure 2-1-2   Simulation diagram of Iliac vein thrombosis

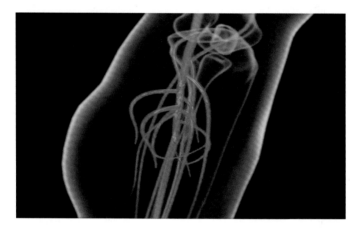

Figure 2-1-3   Simulation diagram of lower extremity deep venous thrombosis

Many risk factors of VTE have been identified by organizations such as the American College of Chest Physicians (ACCP), which has published nine editions of guidelines for VTE diagnosis [3], treatment and prevention from 1995 to 2012. Proposed VTE risk factors include advanced age, infection, malignancy, autoimmune disease, surgery, trauma, pregnancy, long trip syndrome, family history and so on. ACCP has raised the risk stratification of surgical patients. Different measures should be taken in patients with different stratification to prevent VTE. Actually, only a small part of the patients with same risk stratification and same external environment have had VTE. In 2008, Shackfore [4] reported that 84% of the 37619 surgical patients were partly or totally treated and prevented according to the guideline. From 1995, when the first ACCP was published, to 2004, the numbers of symptomatic VTE increased rather than decreased, and there was segregation between preventing risk factors and VTE occurrence.

Thus, here the questions come. Why does the incidence of VTE increase as the age increases? Why does the incidence of VTE stay high in patients with malignancies? Why does only a small part of patients with the same infection develop VTE? Sudden death caused by acute PE resulting from surgeries, pregnancy, delivery or long trip syndrome is always hard to prevent. However, the vast majority of the population will not develop VTE under the same conditions. Both being thrombus, acute arterial thrombus is white thrombus but acute venous thrombus is red thrombus. What does the pathological difference mean? Thrombolytic therapy is effective for arterial thrombosis within several hours after onset, but venous thrombosis, with a wide thrombolytic time window, can be delayed to several days, 2 weeks, or even longer. What causes the difference in the thrombolytic time window between acute venous and acute arterial thrombus? Acute venous thrombus can autolyze, while arterial thrombus cannot. For VTE patients, oral anticoagulants are usually recommended for 3, 6 or 12 months and occasionally life-long. Currently, there are no objective criteria for individual evaluation that complicates the selection of anti-coagulation therapy by physicians. Furthermore, even with standard anti-coagulation therapy and international normalized ratio (INR), some patients still develop CTEPH. Thus, the physicians are extremely puzzled about anticoagulant usage.

Query raised in clinics usually originates from clinical practices. The risk factors of VTE are only the clinical phenomenon of incident VTEs and the summary of evidence-based medicine, not the essence of this disease. So far, the medical resources put into the global prevention of VTE have not had the predicted effects. The reasonable explanation of this separation phenomenon between clinical prevention and treatment guidelines of VTE and clinical practices is that the etiology and pathogenesis of VTE are still unclear.

2. Protein components analysis of acute venous thrombus

The acute venous thrombosis freshly taken out from the body is red to the naked eyes and is fragile. It is composed of red blood cells, platelets, white blood cells and plasma proteins under microscope.

Mass spectrographic analyses have shown that a majority of the proteins in the thrombus are fibrinogen, the the remaining being mainly serum albumin and cytoskeletal proteins [5]. The reversible combinations between the receptor and their ligand-- fibrinogens suggest that acute venous thrombus is easy to autolyze and delayed thrombolysis is effective, so it should be easy to lyse the thrombus through interventional fragmentation.

Acute venous thrombus is red and is composed of red blood cells, platelets, white blood cells and fibrinogen. But how does fibrinogen bind to blood cells in the formation of thrombus? MS/MS and bioinformatics analyses of thrombus in patients with acute PE have shown that subunits β1, β2 and β3 in integrins are the core proteins of acute venous thrombus.

Integrins, important members in cell adhesion molecule family, mediate the adhesion between cells and between cells and extracellular matrix (ECM) and are involved in the bidirectional signaling transduction between cells and ECM. They combine to different ligands in various cellular processes, either physiological or pathological, such as angiogenesis, invasion, metastasis, inflammation, wound healing and coagulation [6].

Integrin is a transmembrane heterodimer composed of subunits α and β at a ratio of 1 : 1. To date, a total of 18 α subunits and 8 β subunits have been identified and they form 24 functional heterodimers, which may be classified into 8 groups (β1-β8) on the basis of β subunit. In the same group, the β subunits are identical but the α subunits are distinct. At rest, the α subunit is covered by the β subunit and thus the integrin is unable to bind to ligands. Following activation, the extension of the β subunit exposes the α subunit. The α subunit mainly mediates the specific and reversible binding between integrins and their ligands, and the β subunit dominates the signal transduction and regulation of affinity of the integrins [7-9].

3. Localization of core proteins in acute venous thrombus

The β1 subunit is mainly found on the lymphocytes and platelets, and its ligand includes laminin, collagen, thrombospondin, fibronetin and VCAM-1. The β2 subunit is mainly distributed on the neutrophils and monocytes, and its ligand includes fibrinogen, ICAM, factor X and ic3b. The β3 subunit is mainly observed on the platelets, and its ligand includes fibrinogen, fibronetin, vitronectin, vWF and thrombospondin [10-12].

In a study, the authors collected the thrombi from patients with acute PE, and detected the expression and distribution of integrins β1, β2 and β3 in thrombi and ligands of integrin subunits β1, β2 and β3 by immunohistochemistry [13]. They found that the dark-brown integrin β1 was expressed on the lymphocytes, but no expression of laminin, fibronectin, collagen-I or collagen-II was observed on the lymphocytes. Meanwhile the dark-brown integrin β2 was expressed on the neutrophils and bound to fibrinogen. ICAM, factor X and iC3b were expressed on neutrophils, whereas the dark-brown integrin β3 was expressed on platelets, which aggregated as a coral-like structure to become thrombotic skeleton, and these platelets bound fibrinogen to construct mesh structure(Figure 2-3-1). No expression of fibronectin, vitronectin or vWF was observed on the platelets; the dark-brown factor Xa was distributed on the mesh-like structure, which was composed of fibrin/fibrinogen.

More than 30 years ago, people invented different types of artificial vena caval filter used in clinics, the mechanism of which is preventing the genesis of PE by blocking the deep venous thrombi flowing back to pulmonary arteries through the filter. Core proteins of thrombi, integrins β2 and β3, bind their ligand fibrinogen to construct mesh structure, which becomes a nest-like filter in thrombi.

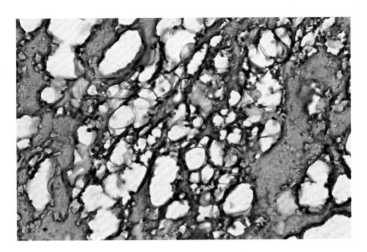

Figure 2-3-1   Immunohistochemistry showed that the dark-brown integrin β3 was expressed on the platlets, which aggregate the skeleton of thrombus and bind with fibrinogen to generate a mesh-like structure (anti-fibrinogen antibody, 1 ∶ 100, ×1000). (International Journal Of Clinical And Experimental Medicine,2015,8(11):19804-19814)

As a precise and perfect life entity, the human body always functions towards the beneficial aspects and the balance, stability and extension of internal and external environments. The construction of intravenous biological filter is the result of self-regulation of human body. But what are the effects of biological filter on human body? And what are the meanings of the body regulation and the construction of a biological filter?

The author of a recent report found a biological filter in veins of the resected sigmoid colon adenocarcinoma tissues [14], in which malignant cells were found in the biological filter and interfered with hematogenous metastasis of cancer cells.

We previously reported virus-like microorganisms in the T lymphocytes of peripheral blood of a PAH and VTE patient with low CD_3 and CD_8 [15] and rod-like bacteria in the phagocytes of peripheral blood in patients with recurrent PE [16]. The heterophilic antigens (pathogenic microorganisms or cancerated cells) cannot be timely or effectively cleared, indicating that the human body needed to build a new defense line when losing functions of immune cells.

4. Inevitability of building a new intravenous defense line

The defense system inside the human body is the immune system. Simply speaking, it is the function of immune system that removes all the foreign agents from human body, including external pathogenic microorganisms, implants, foreign bodies and toxins from wounds, and internal senile cells and malignant cells. Through a long-term evolution, the immune system with both inside and outside functions has developed perfect tissue structures and exceptional functions. The immune system can be divided into innate immune system and adaptive immune system. The innate immunity, also called congenital immunity, is the oldest existing functionality in the biological evolution, which eliminates the encountered foreign bodies immediately through its components, macrophages, granulocytes, natural killer cells and complement system. However, the adaptive immunity, also called specific immunity, is acquired after birth with a characteristic of having memories, which can specifically attack the same invasive foreign agents.

The process of immune balance is a complicated process. When the functions of immune cells blancing collapse, the human body will lose the defensive functions of immune system, external pathogenic microorganisms or tumor cells will intrude into the circulating system, and then the alternative defensive barrier is activated inevitably. It is a basic principle of releasing compensatory reserved functions. The formation of intravenous biological filter indicates the existence of external pathogenic microorganisms or tumor cells in the veins and the supplement of the lost immune functions.

5. Significant downregulation of human immune system related gene mRNA expressions

Human genomics is the study of human genetics with characteristics of wholeness, comprehensiveness and directivity. Although there is difference in the gene-guided protein synthesis among individual proteins, which requires to be validated by proteomic and cytological studies, comparisons of gene expression patterns among different groups and functional analysis of differentially expressed genes may provide a general view and a direction for the understanding of mechanisms underlying the pathogenesis of diseases. This is a unique feature of genomics and cannot be replaced by other methods.

Gene Ontology analysis of the gene expression in PE group targets the significant downregulations of T cell immune complexes and T cell immune functions when compared with the controls [17].

Innate immunity

Phagocytes, NK cells, complement system and cytokine related gene expressions in both PE group and control group were compared.

1) Phagocytes: mRNA expressions of pattern recognition receptors (TLR2, TLR4, CD14, MYD88, MRC1L1, MRC2, MSR1, SCARA5, SCARB2, SCARF1 and SCARF2) and opsonic receptors (CR1, FCGR2A, FCGR2B, FCGR3A and FCGR3B) were up-regulated in phagocytes of the PE group compared with controls, among which TLR4, CD14,

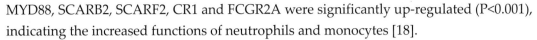

MYD88, SCARB2, SCARF2, CR1 and FCGR2A were significantly up-regulated (P<0.001), indicating the increased functions of neutrophils and monocytes [18].

2) NK cells: Compared with control group, NK cells related gene expressions declined overall in PE group, among which mRNA expressions of seven tenth of the lectin-like receptors and Natural cytotoxic receptors were significantly down-regulated (P<0.05), suggesting reduced functions of NK cells killing target cells directly [18].

3) Complement system: There are 14 genes of complement early components. In PBMCs from PE patients, expression of the genes encoding C1qα, C1qβ, C4b and Factor P was significantly greater (P<0.01) than that in controls. Gene expression of MBL and MASP1 was lower (P<0.05) in PBMCs from PE patients compared with controls, and seven genes of the complement late components were detected. In PE patients, mRNA expression of C5 was significantly up-regulated (P<0.05), whereas C6, C7 and C9 were significantly down-regulated (P<0.05) compared with controls. In PE patients, expression levels of all the seven genes mRNAs were up-regulated, and mRNA expressions of CR1, integrin αM, integrin αX and C5aR were significantly up-regulated (P b 0.01) compared with controls. Gene expressions of complement regulators C4b binding protein, α (C4BPα), C4b binding protein, β (C4BPβ), Factor H, Factor I, CD59, CD55 and CD46 in PBMCs from PE patients and controls were detected. CD59 and CD55 mRNAs were both significantly up-regulated (P<0.05), while Factor I mRNA was significantly down-regulated (P<0.05) in PBMCs from PE patients than controls, and the other 3 genes showed down-regulated trend. mRNA expression of various components, receptors and regulators of the complement pathways were unbalanced in PE patients, indicating the interruption of complement system cascade reactions and the loss of complement mediated membrane attacking functions [19].

4) Cytokines:

a) IFN: In PBMCs from PE patients, the expression levels of genes encoding IFNα5, IFNα6, IFNα8, IFNα14, IFNκ, IFNω1 and IFNϵ1 were significantly lower than those detected in PBMCs from controls (P<0.05). IFNγ mRNA expression was significantly downregulated in PBMCs from PE patients compared with controls (P<0.01) [20].

b) Interleukin genes: A total of 37 interleukin genes were detected. In comparison with the control, the expression levels of 12 genes were downregulated specifically IL1A, IL9, IL17B, IL19, IL23A and IL25 (P<0.05), IL2, IL3, IL13, IL22, IL24 and IL31 (P<0.01), and those of two of the genes, IL10 and IL28A, were upregulated (P<0.05), in the PE patients. The imbalance of Th1/Th2 manifests as reduced cell-mediated immunity [20,21].

c) Chemokines: Twelve genes encoding CXC chemokines were detected. In PE patients, mRNA expression levels of Cxcl1, Cxcl2, Cxcl6, Cxcl13 and Cxcl14 were significantly upregulated (P<0.05), and Cxcl10 mRNA expression levels were significantly downregulated compared with controls (P<0.01). Twenty-three genes encoding CC chemokines were examined and the mRNA expression levels of CC chemokines were significantly lower in PE patients than controls (P<0.01) [20].

d) TNF: Thirty-eight genes encoding members of the TNF superfamily and TNF receptor superfamily were examined. In PE patients, the mRNA expression levels of TNF superfamily members 1, 9 and 13, and TNF receptor superfamily members 1A, 1B, 9, 10B, 10C, 10D and 19L, were significantly upregulated (P<0.05), whereas TNF receptor superfamily members 11B, 19 and 25, were significantly downregulated compared with controls (P<0.05) [20].

e) Colony stimulating factor: Six genes encoding colony stimulating factors were detected and the mRNA expression levels of granulocyte-macrophage colony stimulating factor (GM-CSF), granulocyte colony-stimulating factor (G-CSF), erythropoietin (EPO), thrombopoietin (THPO) and mast cell growth factor (KITLG) were significantly lower in PBMCs from PE patients than controls (P<0.05) [20].

f) Other cytokines: Eight genes associated with transforming growth factor (TGF), epidermal growth factor (EGF) and vascular endothelial growth factor (VEGF) were detected. The mRNA expression levels of TGFβ1, TGFβ1-induced transcript 1, EGF and VEGF were significantly upregulated (P<0.01), whereas TGFβ3 mRNA was significantly downregulated (P<0.05) in PBMCs from PE patients compared with controls [20].

From the characteristics of a variety of cytokine mRNA expression levels in PE patients, we conclude that the immune function and the ability of clearing viruses, intracellular bacteria and parasites are reduced in PE patients [20].

In patients with PE, the expression of the majority of integrin mRNAs located on leukocytes and platelets was significantly upregulated. The expression of mRNAs related to L-selectin and P-selectin glycoprotein ligand was significantly upregulated, while the expression of mRNA related to E-selectin was significantly downregulated. The expression of mRNAs related to classic cadherins and protocadherins was downregulated, and the expression of mRNAs related to vascular endothelial cadherin was significantly downregulated; the expression of mRNAs related to the immunoglobulin superfamily had no obvious difference between the 2 groups. In conclusion, we demonstrated that, in symptomatic PE patients, the adhesion of leukocytes and platelets was enhanced; the activation of endothelial cells was obviously weakened; the adherens junctions among endothelial cells were weakened, with the endothelium becoming more permeable [22].

Among the 13 leukocyte-related integrin mRNAs, integrins β1 and β2 mRNAs expressions were upregulated in the PE group, compared with the controls (P<0.05). Of the 7 platelet-related integrin mRNAs, integrins β2 and β3 mRNAs expressions were upregulated in the PE group, compared with the controls (P<0.05). Among the 11 other integrin mRNAs, 6 were upregulated (of which 3 significantly) in the PE group (P<0.05) and 5 were downregulated (of which 3 significantly) (P<0.01). It can be concluded that

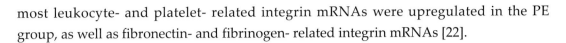

most leukocyte- and platelet- related integrin mRNAs were upregulated in the PE group, as well as fibronectin- and fibrinogen- related integrin mRNAs [22].

Adaptive immunity

T and B lymphocyte related gene expressions in both PE group and control group were compared.

1) T lymphocyte: Of the 6 genes of T cell immunological synapse, receptor complex, plasmalemma and receptors mRNAs, ZAP70, CD247 and GZMB mRNAs were downregulated in the PE group, compared with the controls (P<0.05), while GZMA, CD3G and CD3D mRNAs downregulated in the PE group, compared with the controls (P<0.01) [18].

2) B lymphocyte: mRNA expressions of 82 genes involved in B cell activation were detected.(i)B cell receptor: In PE patients, expressions of LYN, CD22, SYK, BTK, PTPRC and NFAM1 were significantly higher, whereas expressions of FYN, FCRL4 and LAX1 were significantly lower than the control group. (ii)T cell dependent B cell activation: In PE patients, mRNA expressions of EMR2, TNFSF9, CD86, ICOSLG, CD37 and CD97 were significantly up-regulated, whereas SPN mRNA was significantly down-regulated compared with the control group. (iii)T cell independent B cell activation: LILRA1 and TLR9 mRNAs were significantly up-regulated in PE patients compared with the control group. (iv)Regulators: In PE patients, expressions of the genes including CR1, LILRB4 and VAV1 were significantly higher, whereas expression of SLAMF7 was significantly lower than those in the control group. (v) Cytokines: In PE patients, expressions of genes including LTA and IL10 were significantly higher, whereas expressions of L1A, IFNA5, IFNA6, IFNA8, IFNA14, IL2, IL13 and IFNG were significantly lower than those in the control group. It is indicated that Deferential gene expressions in different stages of B cell activation suggest the decrease or disorders of B cell function [23].

The whole genomics results showed significantly decreased functions of T lymphocytes, disorganized functions of B lymphocytes and complements, and inflammations with enhanced immune adherence.

6. DNA sequence mutation in familial VTE patients

We have found that [24], among the familial VTE patients, pore forming protein gene mutations located in NK cells, T cells and complements, were detected in 3 patients with the results of a combined cell deficiency of killing targeted cells. NK cells, CD_8 T cells and complements form the membrane attack complex. The steps of killing foreign or pathological antigen cells include membrane perforation and release of the granzyme. The mutation of pore forming protein gene can lead to membrane perforation function loss. The genomics of symptomatic PE patients showed the significant downregulation of T cell granzyme mRNA expression, which indicates the decreased function of killing cells. Both the mutation and downregulated granzyme mRNA expression suggest the decreased killing activities of immune cells.

7. Immune cell function with VTE

Smeeth [25] reported that the risk for DVT was increased by 1.91 folds within 2 weeks to 6 months after acute infection. In two large case-control studies [26, 27], results also demonstrate that acute infection increases the risk for VTE by 2~3 folds after adjustment of other risk factors of VTE. We found DVTs in multiple organs including pulmonary arteries, kidney, liver and pancreas during autopsy of SARS patient [28], indicating that the genesis of VTE was related to virus infection.

In acute PE [29], the decreased CD_3 and CD_8 levels, and the increased CD_4/CD_8 ratio, were similar to those in CTEPH [30]. We have reported that the functions of CD_3, CD_8, $CD_{16}CD_{56}$ and CD_{19} were compromised or disordered in more than 95% acute symptomatic VTE [31].

T cells are key parts of immune cells, as they regulate the cellular and humoral immunity, and phagocyte functions in innate immunity through Th1, Th2 and Th17. The immune functions decrease when T cell functions decline. The process of immune balance is a complicated process. Different immune functioning status, including normal, decreased and disturbed immune functioning status, decides different body status. The collapse of the balancing functions of immune cells indicates that immune cells in the innate and adaptive systems have a state of no function or dysfunction. We observed significantly decreased T cell functions through cytology, and decreased whole immune cell functions through genomics, indicating the collapse of the balancing functions of immune cells in VTE patients.

8. Malignancy and VTE

Malignancy is one of the risk factors of VTE, and VTE is one of the leading causes of death in patients with malignancy [32-34]. The prevalence of VTE in patients with malignancy is 4-7 times higher than that of patients without malignancy [35, 36].

Malignancy results when cancer cells cannot be effectively and timely cleared by the immune system. The author of a recent study [14] reported that necrosis, granulation tissues, disruption of small veins, and dark brown fibrinogens in veins formed mesh-like structure in sigmoid colon adenocarcinoma. Also, a necrotic region in poorly differentiated gastric carcinoma presented with exudation of a large number of red blood cells. Venous thrombosis and hemorrhage serve as inevitable

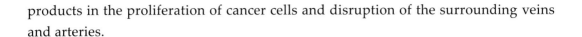

products in the proliferation of cancer cells and disruption of the surrounding veins and arteries.

9. Expression of same / different proteins in venous thromboembolism and different risk factor group patients

In a previous study [38], we recruited a total of 1006 subjects and divided them into VTE group, risk factor groups and control (non- risk factor) group without a difference in age. Flow cytometry was performed to detect the expression of the core proteins in venous thrombi. The normal range of integrins β1, β2 and β3 were generated from healthy people.

Compared with that in the control group, the integrin β1 expression in VTE group and subjects with different risk factors (acute infection, malignancy and autoimmune diseases) increased markedly (P<0.001, <0.01). However, compared with the control group, the integrin β1 expression in trauma /surgery group was not significantly different (P>0.05). The elevated expression of integrin β1 in VTE group, acute infection group, malignancy group and autoimmune diseases group was highly consistent with the increased core protein expression in thrombi, indicating that VTE patients shared the same protein expression with patients with acute infection, malignancy and autoimmune diseases. However, similar elevations of protein expression were not found in patients with trauma /surgery.

Compared with the control group, the integrin β2 expression in VTE group increased significantly (P <0.05). However, compared with control group, the integrin β2 expression in subjects with different risk factors (acute infection, malignancy and autoimmune diseases,trauma /surgery group) was not significantly different (P>0.05), suggesting no same elevation of protein expression was found in patients with acute infection group, malignancy group and autoimmune diseases group, trauma /surgery group.

Compared with control group, the integrin β3 expression in VTE group was elevated (P<0.05). However, the integrin β3 expression in different risk factor groups (acute infection, malignancy, autoimmune diseases, trauma/ surgery) were not significantly different (P>0.05).

We found that integrins β2 and β3 are the proteins to distinguish patient with VTE from patients with risk factors, and are also the key proteins for determining the occurrence of VTE. The increased integrin β1 is the characterized expression in patients with risk factors. However this increased expression of integrins β1, β2 and β3 was not found in patients following trauma or surgery, calling into question that such patients may have no VTE risk.

10. Core proteins may serve as new specific protein markers for VTE diagnosis

The author of a report [39] adopted ROC curve analysis to assess diagnostic performance of these core proteins in 120 VTE patients. When a comparison was made between VTE patients and non-VTE patients plus healthy controls, the AUC of integrin β1, integrin β2 and integrin β3 was 0.870, 0.821 and 0.731, respectively. Optimum cutoffs of integrin β1, integrin β2 and integrin β3 calculated according to Youden's index were 10.29pg/ml, 91.10pg/ml and 10.35pg/ml, respectively. With these optimum cutoffs, the sensitivity, specificity, positive predictive value and negative predictive value of integrin β1 were 80.3%, 83.7%, 71.1% and 89.3%, respectively; integrin β2 78.6%, 73.7%, 59.4% and 87.6%; integrin β3 68.4%, 71.2%, 54.3% and 81.8%. The AUC of combined three integrins was 0.916, the sensitivity, specificity, positive predictive value and negative predictive value were 84.6%, 90.8%, 81.7% and 92.0%, respectively. Clinical researches have confirmed significantly increased expression of integrins β1, β2 and β3 in VTE patients, which had relatively high specificity and sensitivity.

Taken together, with underlying conditions of collapsed immune cell balancing function, cells infected by pathogenic microorganisms and malignant cells may trigger intravenous immune adhesive inflammation, which is the defensive reaction in human body to establish the intravenous biological filter preventing infected cells and malignant cells from flowing back. However, the red thrombus forms and the defense transfers into thrombotic disease, when the filter is filled with red blood cells.

People with collapsed immune cell balancing functions are the vulnerable groups for venous thromboembolism. In a patient of venous thromboembolism, it is very possible that the genesis of venous thrombosis was triggered by infected cells or malignant cells. Only under the condition of immune cell balancing function collapse, the risk factors, such as advanced age, infection, malignancy, autoimmune disease, pregnancy, long trip syndrome, as well as family history may cause venous thrombosis. However, even with definable risk factors, there is no risk of getting venous thromboembolism in patients without collapsed immune cell balancing function.

Core proteins in acute venous thrombus are integrins β1, β2 and β3. The increased integrin β1 is the characterized expression in people with risk factors of VTE. However this increased expression of integrins β1, β2 and β3 was not found in patients following trauma or surgery calling into question that such patients may have no VTE risk. Therefore, trauma or surgery may be not the "true" risk factor for VTE.

It should be extended to the upstream of the disease from the middle and lower reaches to prevent the VTE, to decrease the incidence and to increase the cure rate. Hence, it is not enough only to prevent and reduce the known risk factors. Rather, the adjustment and improvement of immune cell balancing function, lowering the stress level inside human body, and restoring the balance of neuroendocrine functions, are new contents of prevention, treatment and rehabilitation of VTE.

(Published: Int J Clin Exp Med 2015;8(11):19804-19814)

References

1. Piazza G and Goldhaber SZ. Physician alerts to prevent venous thromboembolism. J Thromb Thrombolysis 2010; 30: 1-6.

2. Prevention and treatment of venous thromboembolism. International Consensus Statement (guidelines according to scientific evidence). Int Angiol 2006; 25: 101-161.

3. Guyatt GH, Akl EA, Crowther M, Gutterman DD and Schuunemann HJ. Executive summary: Antithrombotic Therapy and Prevention of Thrombosis, 9th ed: American College of Chest Physicians Evidence-Based Clinical Practice Guidelines. Chest 2012; 141: 7s-47s.

4. Shackford SR, Rogers FB, Terrien CM, Bouchard P, Ratliff J and Zubis R. A 10-year analysis of venous thromboembolism on the surgical service: the effect of practice guidelines for prophylaxis. Surgery 2008; 144: 3-11.

5. Wang L, Gong Z, Jiang J, Xu W, Duan Q, Liu J and Qin C. Confusion of wide thrombolytic time window for acute pulmonary embolism: mass spectrographic analysis for thrombus proteins. Am J Respir Crit Care Med 2011; 184: 145-146.

6. Giancotti FG and Ruoslahti E. Integrin signaling. Science 1999; 285: 1028-1032.

7. Humphries MJ. Integrin structure. Biochem Soc Trans 2000; 28: 311-339.

8. Takada Y, Ye X and Simon S. The integrins. Genome Biol 2007; 8: 215.

9. Xiong JP, Stehle T, Diefenbach B, Zhang R, Dunker R, Scott DL, Joachimiak A, Goodman SL and Arnaout MA. Crystal structure of the extracellular segment of integrin alpha Vbeta3. Science 2001; 294: 339-345.

10. Solovjov DA, Pluskota E and Plow EF. Distinct roles for the alpha and beta subunits in the functions of integrin alphaMbeta2. J Biol Chem 2005; 280: 1336-1345.

11. Gerber DJ, Pereira P, Huang SY, Pelletier C and Tonegawa S. Expression of alpha v and beta 3 integrin chains on murine lymphocytes. Proc Natl Acad Sci U S A 1996; 93: 14698-14703.

12. Litynska A, Przybylo M, Ksiazek D and Laidler P. Differences of alpha3beta1 integrin glycans from different human bladder cell lines. Acta Biochim Pol 2000; 47: 427-434.

13. Wang LM, Duan QL, Yang F, Yi XH, Zeng Y, Tian HY, Lv W and Jin Y. Activation of circulated immune cells and inflammatory immune adherence are involved in the whole process of acute venous thrombosis. Int J Clin Exp Med 2014; 7: 566-572.

14. Wang LM, Duan QL, Yi XH, Zeng Y, Gong Z and Yang F. Venous thromboembolism is a product in proliferation of cancer cells. Int J Clin Exp Med 2014; 7: 1319-1323.

15. Wang L, Gong Z, Liang A, Xie Y, Liu SL, Yu Z, Wang L and Wang Y. Compromised T-cell immunity and virus-like structure in a patient with pulmonary hypertension. Am J Respir Crit Care Med 2010; 182: 434-435.

16. Wang LM, Zhang XY, Duan QL, Lv W, Gong Z, Xie Y, Liang AB and Wang Y. Rod-like bacteria and recurrent venous thromboembolism. Am J Respir Crit Care Med 2012; 186: 696.

17. Wang H, Duan Q, Wang L, Gong Z, Liang A, Wang Q, Song H, Yang F and Song Y. Analysis on the pathogenesis of symptomatic pulmonary embolism with human genomics. Int J Med Sci 2012; 9: 380-386.

18. Gong Z, Liang AB, Wang LM, et al. The expression andsignificance of immunity associated genes mRNA in patients withpulmonary embolism [in Chinese]. Zhonghua Nei Ke Za Zhi 2009;48:666-669.

19. Lv W, Wang L, Duan Q, Gong Z, Yang F, Song H and Song Y. Characteristics of the complement system gene expression deficiency in patients with symptomatic pulmonary embolism. Thromb Res 2013; 132: e54-57.

20. Lv W, Duan Q, Wang L, Gong Z, Yang F and Song Y. Gene expression levels of cytokines in peripheral blood mononuclear cells from patients with pulmonary embolism. Mol Med Rep 2013; 7: 1245-1250.

21. Duan Q, Lv W, Wang L, Gong Z, Wang Q, Song H and Wang H. mRNA expression of interleukins and Th1/Th2 imbalance in patients with pulmonary embolism. Mol Med Rep 2013; 7: 332-336.

22. Xie Y, Duan Q, Wang L, Gong Z, Wang Q, Song H and Wang H. Genomic characteristics of adhesion molecules in patients with symptomatic pulmonary embolism. Mol Med Rep 2012; 6: 585-590.

23. Lv W, Duan Q, Wang L, Gong Z, Yang F and Song Y. Expression of B-cell-associated genes in peripheral blood mononuclear cells of patients with symptomatic pulmonary embolism. Mol Med Rep 2015; 11: 2299-2305.

24. Qianglin Duan,Wei Lv, Minjun Yang, Fan Yang, Yongqiang Zhu, Hui Kang, Haoming Song, Shengyue Wang, Lemin Wang, Hui Dong Characterization of immune cells and perforin mutations in a family with venous thromboembolism Int J Clin Exp Med 2015;8(5):7951-7957

25. Smeeth L, Cook C, Thomas S, Hall AJ, Hubbard R and Vallance P. Risk of deep vein thrombosis and pulmonary embolism after acute infection in a community setting. Lancet 2006; 367: 1075-1079.

26. Clayton TC, Gaskin M and Meade TW. Recent respiratory infection and risk of venous thromboembolism: case-control study through a general practice database. Int J Epidemiol 2011; 40: 819-827.

27. Schmidt M, Horvath-Puho E, Thomsen RW, Smeeth L and Sorensen HT. Acute infections and venous thromboembolism. J Intern Med 2012; 271: 608-618.

28. Yi XH, Wang LM, Liang AB, Gong Z, Lai RQ, Zhu XY, Rui WW and Wang YN. Severe acute respiratory syndrome and venous thromboembolism in multiple organs. Am J Respir Crit Care Med 2010; 182: 436-437.

29. Wang L, Song H, Gong Z, Duan Q and Liang A. Acute pulmonary embolism and dysfunction of CD_3 CD_8 T cell immunity. Am J Respir Crit Care Med 2011; 184: 1315.

30. Song HM, Wang LM, Gong Z, Liang AB, Xie Y, Lv W, Jiang JF, Xu WJ and Shen YQ. T cell-mediated immune deficiency or compromise in patients with CTEPH. Am J Respir Crit Care Med 2011; 183: 417-418.

31. Duan Q, Gong Z, Song H, Wang L, Yang F, Lv W and Song Y. Symptomatic venous thromboembolism is a disease related to infection and immune dysfunction. Int J Med Sci 2012; 9: 453-461.

32. Chew HK, Wun T, Harvey D, Zhou H, White RH. Incidence of venous thromboembolism and its effect on survival among patients with common cancers. Archives of Internal Medicine 2006;166:458-64.

33. Khorana AA, Liebman HA, White RH, Wun T and Lyman GH. The risk of venous thromboembolism in patients with cancer. Ame Society of Clin Oncol Educ Book 2008; 240-248.

34. Chew HK, Wun T, Harvey DJ, Zhou H, White RH. Incidence of venous thromboembolism and the impact on survival in breast cancer patients. Journal of Clinical Oncology 2007;25:70-6.

35. Wun T and White RH. Epidemiology of cancer-related venous thromboembolism. Best Prac Res Clin Haematol 2009; 22: 9-23.

36. Blom JW, Doggen CJ, Osanto S and Rosendaal FR. Malignancies, prothrombotic mutations, and the risk of venous thrombosis. Jama 2005; 293: 715-722.

37. Le-Min Wang, Qiang-Lin Duan, Xiang-Hua Yi, Yu Zeng, Zhu Gong, Fan Yang. Venous thromboembolism is a product in proliferation of cancer cells. Int J Clin Exp Med 2014; 7: 1319-1323.

38. Duan Q, Wang L, Yang F, Li J, SongY, Gong Z, Li G, Song H, Zhang X, Shen Z, Dart A. Internal relationship between symptomatic venous thromboembolism and risk factors: up-regulation of integrin β1, β2 and β3 levels. Am J Transl Res 2015; 7(3):624-631.

39. Song Y, Yang F, Wang L, Duan Q, Jin Y and Gong Z. Increased expressions of integrin subunit beta1, beta2 and beta3 in patients with venous thromboembolism: new markers for venous thromboembolism. Int J Clin Exp Med 2014; 7: 2578-2584.

Chapter 3

Components of acute venous red thrombus

1. Pathology of acute venous thrombus

Acute venous thrombus is characterized by easy degradation and autolysis. Delayed thrombolysis is effective on acute massive pulmonary embolism (PE); usually only low molecular heparin is used to dissolve thrombus in submassive PE. Interventional fragmentation is adopted to quickly lyse the massive thrombus and effectively recover the blood flow in the pulmonary artery when thrombolysis is contraindicated in patients with acute massive PE. However, the arterial thrombus lacks this kind of characteristics.

Acute venous thrombus is red thrombus, which is composed of red blood cells, platelets, white blood cells and plasma proteins under the microscope (Figure 3-1-1).

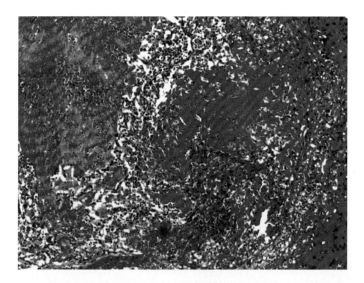

Figure 3-1-1　HE staining of venous thrombus. It is red thrombus, in which massive red blood cells and white blood cells with dark-brown nuclei are aggregated (HE staining, ×200). (International Journal Of Clinical And Experimental Medicine , 2015 , 8 (11) : 19804-19814)

2. Main protein components of acute venous thrombus

Although the principle in the treatment of venous and arterial thrombosis is identical, the thrombolytic time window differs largely. Thrombolytic therapy is effective within several hours after onset for arterial thrombosis but as long as several days, two weeks or even longer for venous thrombosis. The mechanism underlying the difference in the thrombolytic time window between venous and arterial thromboses still remains unclear.

Pulmonary artery catheter angiography was performed in a 31-year-old patient who got dyspnea without any definite cause and PE diagnosis was confirmed. The catheter was inserted to the pulmonary artery, and the embolus was obtained for mass spectrographic analysis of thrombus proteins. Results showed that a majority of proteins were less than 130 kDa with great differences in abundance. The proteins with the relative abundance of trace to 34.34% could be observed (Figure 3-2-1).

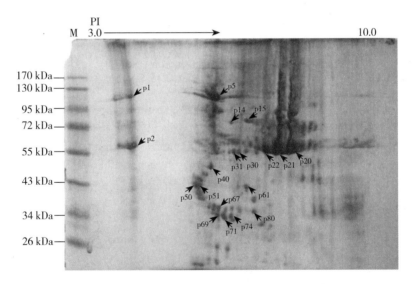

Figure 3-2-1   Electrophoresis of thrombus proteins of an acute PE patient. The mass spectrographic analysis results are summarized in Table 3-2-1. (American Journal Of Respiratory And Critical Care Medicine,2011,184: 145-146)

Mass spectrographic analyses showed that a majority of the proteins were fibrinogen, and the remaining included serum albumin and cytoskeletal proteins.

Early thrombolytic therapy may bring favorable effects [1-3]. Furthermore, some patients can benefit from thrombolytic therapy even 6~14 days after PE [4]. In our experience, when the thrombolytic therapy was applied in patients more than 2 weeks after PE, favorable outcome could still be achieved, although the mechanism underlying

Table 3-2-1   The components of thrombus proteins

Protein name	PI	MW	Content (%)	Characterization	Pub med No.
p1	5.54	46252	0.38	fibrinogen gamma/Fibrinogen is involved in blood clotting, being activated by thrombin to assemble into fibrin clots	0602239A
p2	7.14	52281	1.42	Chain B, Crystal Structure Of Human Fibrinogen	3GHG_B
p5	5.54	46438	7.08	Chain C, Crystal Structure Of Human Fibrinogen	3GHG_C
p14	5.63	65778	0.16	Chain A, Structure Of Human Serum Albumin With S-Naproxen And The Ga Module	2VDB_A
p15	8.54	55892	0.75	fibrinogen, beta chain preproprotein	NP_005132
p20	8.31	54861	34.34	beta-fibrinogen precursor	AAA52429
p21	8.54	55892	31.92	fibrinogen, beta chain preproprotein	NP_005132
p22	8.54	55892	5.37	fibrinogen, beta chain preproprotein	NP_005132
p30	6.95	39711	0.26	fibrinogen beta chain, isoform CRA_e	EAX04934
p31	5.84	37625	0.43	Chain B, Crystal Structure Of Fibrinogen Fragment D	1FZA_B
p40	5.37	41738	0.56	beta actin variant/An ubiquitous protein involved in the formation of filaments that are a major component of the cytoskeleton. Interaction with myosin provides the basis of muscular contraction and many aspects of cell motility	BAD96752
p50	5.54	46252	0.38	fibrinogen gamma	0602239A
p51	5.54	46438	0.45	Chain C, Crystal Structure Of Human Fibrinogen	3GHG_C
p61	8.33	52131	0.42	fibrinogen beta chain, isoform CRA_d [Homo sapiens]	EAX04933
p67	5.54	46252	0.28	fibrinogen gamma	0602239A
p69	5.54	46252	0.37	fibrinogen gamma	0602239A
p71	5.54	46252	0.64	fibrinogen gamma	0602239A
p74	6.49	24109	0.44	fibrinogen gamma chain	CAA35837
p80	8.33	52131	0.35	fibrinogen beta chain, isoform CRA_d [Homo sapiens]	EAX04933

26

the wide thrombolytic time window in PE patients remains unclear. According to the phlebothrombosis theory, in veins the blood flow is slow, and the thrombus is rich in fibrin and red cells, only with a small amount of platelets. Ten days after the onset of acute PE, the embolus was found to be red embolus, flexible, elastic, and fragile. Our mass spectrographic analysis showed that the main component of thrombus in acute PE was fibrinogen, with some serum albumin and cytoskeletal proteins. Fibrinogen makes the embolus fragile, which explains the reason of wide thrombolytic time window and also explains why PE patients with stable hemodynamics may benefit from anticoagulant therapy alone, and interventional thromboclasis is still effective for acute PE patients [5]. The thrombus of VTE in pathology mainly includes red thrombus and mixed thrombus, with a small mount of white thrombus. The protein component of red thrombus in acute PE is mainly fibrinogen, which can convert to fibrin, but this needs some time. This change needing the time may explain why VTE patients may benefit from anticoagulant therapy alone and the reason of wide thrombolytic time window.

(Published: Am J Respir Crit Care Med 2011;184:145-6.)

References

1. Urokinase pulmonary embolism trial. Phase 1 results: a cooperative study. JAMA. 1970 Dec 21;214(12):2163-72.

2. Goldhaber SZ, Haire WD, Feldstein ML, Miller M, Toltzis R, Smith JL, et al. Alteplase versus heparin in acute pulmonary embolism: randomised trial assessing right-ventricular function and pulmonary perfusion. Lancet. 1993;341:507-11.

3. Goldhaber SZ, Kessler CM, Heit JA, Elliott CG, Friedenberg WR, Heiselman DE, et al. Recombinant tissue-type plasminogen activator versus a novel dosing regimen of urokinase in acute pulmonary embolism: a randomized controlled multicenter trial. J Am Coll Cardiol. 1992;20:24-30.

4. Daniels LB, Parker JA, Patel SR, Grodstein F, Goldhaber SZ. Relation of duration of symptoms with response to thrombolytic therapy in pulmonary embolism. Am J Cardiol. 1997;80:184-8.

5. Wang L, Wei L, Liu Y, Li X, Guo X, Zhi J, et al. Optional therapeutic strategies based on clinically different types of acute pulmonary embolism. Chin Med J (Engl). 2003;116:849-52.

3. Core proteins in acute venous thrombus

In 2011, we reported that the main protein component of red venous thrombus in APE was fibrinogen, rather than fibrin, with only a small quantity of cellular cytoskeletal and plasma proteins [1].

The report explained why the delayed thrombolytic therapy and thrombus fragmentation through a catheter are effective for acute VTE. However, the location and distribution of fibrinogen in thrombosis remain unclear. In addition, it has been reported that the use of antiplatelet drug aspirin alone for prevention and treatment of VTE cannot achieve good outcomes [2], suggesting that the role of platelets in the occurrence of VTE needs to be re-clarified.

Pathologically, there is mainly red venous thrombus in acute VTE, being composed of erythrocytes, platelets, leukocytes and proteins such as fibrinogen. Fibrinogen is a key protein in the coagulation system, and it consists of a symmetrical heterodimer. The binding of fibrinogen to leukocytes and platelets in the venous thrombus is involved in the pathogenesis of venous thrombus. We hypothesized that, due to the binding of fibrinogens (ligands) and activated receptors on the surfaces of leukocytes, platelets and lymphocytes, the thrombus protein network is constructed and red venous thrombus forms with erythrocytes and plasma components being filled in the protein network spaces.

Collection of acute VTE thrombus

Several 5-15mm red venous thrombi weighing 10-20 g were extracted from the pulmonary artery of 4 male patients (39, 45, 50, 61 years) with APE and the femoral vein of a 50-year-old male by femoral venous puncturing using a 7F catheter (Metronic USA). Tandem mass spectrometry was performed for 2 cases, and pathological analysis was performed for the other 3 cases.

Tandem mass spectrometry [3]

Acute PE thrombi-MS/MS (LTQ, Thermo Finnigan USA) (sample preparation, sample pre-isolation Figure 3-3-1 (left), peptide segment enzymolysis and fragment sequence data Figure 3-3-1 (right))-database-retrieve proteins - corresponding genes-Gene Ontology analysis - differential genes - differential proteins - KEGGPathway-

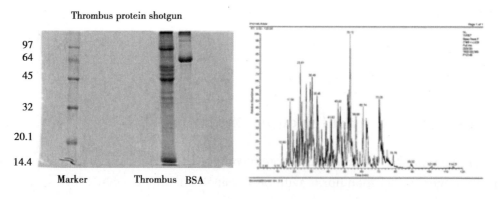

Figure 3-3-1   Component analysis of thrombus. Left: Thrombus pre-isolation of acute thrombus; right: MS/MS fragment sequence information of acute thrombus.

geneNetwork - the core proteins of the thrombus protein network.

The data on peptides following tandem mass spectrometry were subjected to bioinformatics analysis, the proteins corresponding to peptides were precisely determined, and the corresponding genes were searched.

Gene network analysis

The ways in which interaction is performed were integrated from 1) the KEGG database in which protein interaction, gene regulation and protein modification are shown [4]; 2) the studies with high throughout detection; 3) studies reporting the interaction among genes. The pathways in KEGG database were employed to analyze the interaction among genes with a software from KEGGSOAP [5] (http://www. bioconductor.org/packages/2.4/bioc/html/KEGGSOAP.html), including the following three relationships:

ECrel: enzyme-enzyme relation, indicating two enzymes catalyzing successive reaction steps; PPrel: protein-protein interaction, such as binding and modification.

GErel: gene expression interaction, indicating relation of transcription factor and target gene product.

The interaction among genes is not confined to a specific pathway, which is different from the KEGG-Pathway database. On the pathways in which gene interaction acts, the downstream and upstream genes of screened genes are searched. The overlapping genes between screened genes and their downstream and upstream genes are further analyzed, and the pathways in which screened genes interact with other genes are identified. The genes are symbolized with circle which is then marked with different colors depending on the up-regulation/down-regulation, difference/ non-difference. One or more pathways may be present and expressed with lines characterized by arrows with different shapes. Binding among proteins: two proteins bind to form a complex, which has no direction and a line without arrow is used. Binding induced activation leading to increase in expression: protein A may activate the gene transcription of protein B leads to the increase in gene expression, which has a direction and is expressed with an arrowheaded line. Activation: protein A may activate the functions of protein B via interaction, which has a direction and is expressed with an arrowheaded line. Inhibition: protein A may inhibit the functions of protein B via interaction, which has a direction and is expressed with a "T" shaped line.

Results

Informatics showed that the core proteins were integrins in the protein network of embolus of APE (Figure 3-3-2).

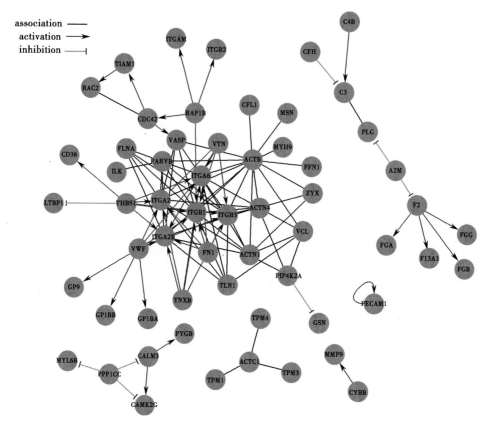

Figure 3-3-2 MS/MS and bioinformatics analysis of embolus in patients with acute PE. Subunits β1, β2 and β3 in integrins were the core proteins of embolus. (International Journal Of Clinical And Experimental Medicine,2015,8(11):19804-19814)

Discussion

Venous red thrombus is constituted by coralline skeleton and fibrinogenic filamentous sieve to possess the function of biological venous filter. The filter is filled with blood cells, mainly erythrocytes, so red thrombus is formed. Our findings demonstrate that the subunits β1, β2 and β3 in integrins are the core proteins of the network of venous red thrombi. In the red thrombi, β1 is localized on the platelets and lymphocytes, β2 is mainly found on the leucocytes and β3 is predominantly observed on the platelets. Results from bioinformatics analysis are consistent with those from immunohistochemistry. Integrins are important members in cell adhesion molecule family and mediate the adhesion between cells and between cells and extracellular matrix (ECM).

Integrin is a transmembrane heterodimer composed of subunits α and β at a ratio of 1 : 1. To date, a total of 18 α subunits and 8 β subunits have been identified and they can form 24 functional heterodimers which may be classified into 8 groups (β1-β8) on the basis of β subunit. In the same group, the β subunit is identical, but the α subunit is distinct. At rest, the α subunit is covered by the β subunit and thus the integin is unable to bind to ligands. Following activation, the extension of the β subunit exposes the α subunit. The α subunit mainly mediates the specific and reversible binding between integrins and their ligands, and the β subunit dominates the signal transduction and regulation of affinity of integrins [6,7,8] (Figure 3-3-3,4,5).

The β1 subunit is mainly found on the lymphocytes and platelets, and its ligands include laminin, collagen, thrombospondin, fibronetin and VCAM-1 [6,7]. The β2 subunit is mainly distributed on the neutrophils and monocytes, and its ligands include fibrinogen, ICAM, factorX and ic3b [6,7,10,11]. The β3 subunit is mainly observed on the platelets, and its ligands include fibrinogen, fibronetin, vitronectin, vWF and

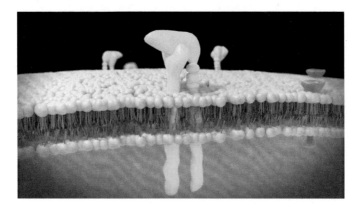

Figure 3-3-3   Integrin is a transmembrane heterodimer formed by one α subunit and one β subunit via a non-covalent bond. At resting state, α subunit does not bind to its ligand. (International Journal Of Clinical And Experimental Medicine,2015,8(11):19804-19814)

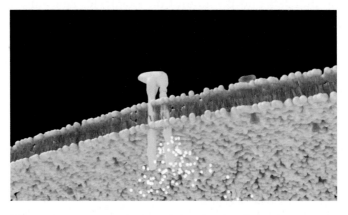

Figure 3-3-4   α subunit and β subunit of an integrin are regulated by extracellular signals

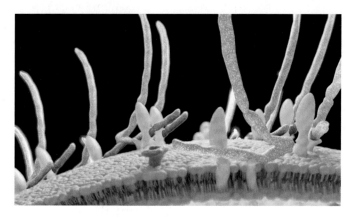

Figure 3-3-5   Following integrin activation, α subunit departs
from β subunit and binds to its ligand.

thrombospondin [6,7,12].

The activated integrins in β1, β2 and β3 groups can bind to corresponding ligands via the α subunit, mediating the adhesion between cells and between cells and ECM.

From the receptor and ligand relationship, β1 intergrins mediate the homing of lymphocytes, intercellular adhesion and adhesion between cells and matrix protein, and also mediate the adhesion between platelets and blood vessel endothelium. β2 integrins mediate adhesion between cells and matrix protein. β3 intergrins mediate the aggregation of platelets and the adhesion of platelets to the basement membrane involving in thrombosis. The formation of venous red thrombus can be explained as a process of adhesion between receptors and corresponding ligands on cells. Two receptors on platelets bind to one ligand fibrinogen in a β3 dependent manner leading to the aggregation of platelets [13-16], and the skeleton of thrombus is formed. The results suggest that the platelets aggregated to become the skeleton structure of a thrombus. The β3 subunit on platelets and β2 subunit on leucocytes can bind to the fibrinogen, forming a filamentous sieve in which blood cells are filled. The skeleton structure and the filamentous sieve lead to the formation of biological venous filter. The main protein of thrombus is fibrinogen, the receptor of which is β3 intergrin. The platelets aggregated coralline skeleton structure and the filamentous sieve are both related to β3 intergrins. So, integrin β3 plays important roles in venous thrombosis. We have found the reason why the antiplatelet drug aspirin alone for prevention and treatment of VTE cannot achieve good outcomes, which is because aspirin binds to different receptors of platelets, not β1 or β3 receptors.

Bioinformatics analysis was employed to analyze the data from tandem mass spectrometry of proteins in thrombi, and the core proteins in thrombi were determined.

References

1. Wang L, Gong Z, Jiang J, Xu W, Duan Q, Liu J,Qin C. Confusion of wide thrombolytic time window for acute pulmonary embolism: mass spectrographic analysis for thrombus proteins. Am J Respir Crit Care Med. 2011; 184:145-146.

2. Watson HG, Chee YL. Aspirin and other antiplatelet drugs in the prevention of venous thromboembolism. Blood Rev. 2008;22(2):107-16.

3. Jin WH, Dai J, Li SJ, Xia QC, Zou HF, Zeng R. Human plasma proteome analysis by multidimensional chromatography prefractionation and linear ion trap mass spectrometry identification. J Proteome Res. 2005; 4(2):613-9.

4. Kanehisa M, Goto S, Furumichi M, Tanabe M, Hirakawa M. KEGG for representation and analysis of molecular networks involving diseases and drugs. Nucleic Acids Res. 2010;38(Database issue):D355-60.

5. Antonov AV, Schmidt EE, Dietmann S, Krestyaninova M, Hermjakob H. R spider: a network-based analysis of gene lists by combining signaling and metabolic pathways from Reactome and KEGG databases. Nucleic Acids Res. 2010;38(Web Server issue):W78-83.

6. Takada Y, Ye X, Simon S. The integrins. Genome Biol. 2007;8(5):215.

7. Var der Flier A, Sonnenberg A. Functions and integrins. Cell and tissue research.2001;305:285-298.

8. Xiong JP, Stehle T, Diefenbach B, et al.Crystal structure of the extracellular segment of integrin alpha Vbeta3. Science. 2001; 294(5541):339-45.

9. Humphries MJ. Integrin structure. Biochem Soc Trans. 2000; 28(4):311-39.

10. Solovjov DA, Pluskota E, Plow EF. Distinct roles for the alpha and beta subunits in the functions of integrin alphaMbeta2. J Biol Chem. 2005; 280(2):1336-45.

11. Gerber DJ, Pereira P, Huang SY, Pelletier C, Tonegawa S. Expression of alpha v and beta 3 integrin chains on murine lymphocytes. Proc Natl Acad Sci U S A. 1996; 93(25):14698-703.

12. Lityńska A, Przybyło M, Ksiazek D, Laidler P. Differences of alpha3beta1 integrin glycans from different human bladder cell lines. Acta Biochim Pol. 2000; 47(2):427-34.

13. Hughes PE, Pfaff M. Integrin affinity modulation. Trends Cell Biol. 1998 Sep;8(9):359-64.

14. Kasirer-Friede A, Kahn ML, Shattil SJ. Platelet integrins and immunoreceptors. Immunol Rev, 2007;218: 247-264.

15. Mendolicchio GL, Ruggeri ZM. New perspectives on von Willebrand factor functions in hemostasis and thrombosis. Semin Hematol, 2005; 42(1): 5-14.

16. Quinn MJ, Byzova TV, Qin J, et al. Integrin alphaIIbbeta3 and its antagonism. Arterioscler Thromb Vasc Biol, 2003; 23(6): 945-952.

4. The inflammatory immune adherence is involved in the whole process of acute venous thrombosis

We have reported that the main component of acute venous thrombi is fibrinogen

[1]. In our previous study, the thrombi were collected from patients with acute PE, and tandem mass spectrometry and bioinformatics were employed to determine that integrin subunit β1, β2 and β3 are core proteins of acute venous thrombi. Immunohistochemistry was performed to investigate the expression and cell distribution of integrins β1, β2 and β3 in acute venous thrombi and the binding with different ligands in these cells. We aimed to explore the role of immune cells in the process of acute venous thrombosis.

Samples

Thrombi (n=5-8; 5-15 mm in length and 10-20 g in weight) were collected from the pulmonary artery of a patient with acute PE and samples were prepared for pathological examination.

Immunohistochemistry and observation under a light microscope

After preparation of thrombus samples, HE staining, immunohistochemistry and Masson staining were performed. The following reagents were used in this study: integrin β1 : 1 : 50 (abcam B3B11), integrin β2 : 1 : 150 (abcam MEM-48), integrin β3 : 1 : 150 (abcam PM6/13); ligand anti-Laminin antibody 1 : 50 (abcam14055), ligand anti-Fibronectin antibody 1 : 50 (abcam2413), ligand anti-Collagen I antibody 1 : 50 (abcam34710), ligand anti-Collagen II antibody 1 : 50 (abcam34712), ligand anti-fibrinogen antibody1 : 100 (abcam ab34269), ligand anti-Factor X antibody1 : 50 (abcam ab11871), ligand anti-Factor Xa heavy chain antibody 1 : 50 (abcam ab140112), ligand anti-C3/C3b antibody1 : 50 (abcam ab11871), ligand anti-ICAM1 antibody 1 : 50 (abcam124759), ligand Von Willebrand Factor antibody 1 : 50 (abcam11713), ligand anti-Vitronectin antibody1 : 50 (abcam28023).

Results

(1) Acute venous thrombi were red thrombi in which there are cord-like structures, and the spaces were filled with a large amount of aggravated red blood cells and nucleated blood cells (Figure 3-4-1).

(2) Immunohistochemistry showed that integrin β1 was expressed on the lymphocytes (Figure 3-4-2A), but no expression of Laminin, Fibronectin, Collagen I or Collagen-II (receptors of integrin β1) was observed on the lymphocytes (Figure 3-4-2B, C, D, E).

(3) Immunohistochemistry showed that integrin β2 was expressed on the neutrophils (Figure 3-4-3A), which bound to fibrinogen (Figure3-4-3B). The ICAM, factor X and iC3b were expressed on neutrphils (Figure 3-4-3C, D, E).

(4) Immunohistochemistry showed that integrin β3 was expressed on platelets, which aggregated to be thrombotic skeleton (Figure 3-4-4A) and coral-like structure

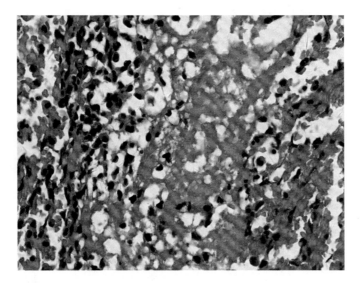

Figure 3-4-1   HE staining of thrombus shows that the venous thrombus is red thrombus, in which cord-like structures, massive red blood cells and white blood cells with dark-brown nuclei aggregated (HE staining, ×400). (International Journal Of Clinical And Experimental Medicine,2014,7: 566-572)

(Figure 3-4-4B); these platelets bound fibrinogen to construct mesh structure (Figure 3-4-4C). No expression of Fibronectin, Vitronectin or vWF was observed on the platelets (Figure 3-4-4D, E, F).

(5) The thrombi had mesh-like structure (Figure 3-4-5A, Masson staining), in which a large amount of red blood cell dominant blood cells filled (Figure 3-4-5C, Masson staining). In colon cancer tissues, there are widely distributed dark-brown mesh-like structures in the venules (Figure 3-4-5B anti-fibrinogen antibody1:100), in which a variety of cancer cells filled (Figure 3-4-5D).

(6) Dark-brown Factor Xa was distributed on the mesh-like structure, which was composed of fibrin/fibrinogen (Figure 3-4-6A, B).

The integrin family was initially recognized as adhesion molecules mediating the adhesion between cells and extracellular matrix, which leads to the integration of cells. Integrins are widely distributed in human body. A kind of integrin can be distributed in a variety of types of cells, and one cell may have the expression of several integrins. The expression of integrins varies from activation status and differentiation status of cells [2]. Integrin is a transmembrane heterodimer composed of α and β subunits at a ratio of 1:1 via the non-covalent bond. A total of 8 β subunits (β1-β8) have been identified in human. Under the quiescent condition, the β subunit covers the α subunit, and thus the integrin fails to bind ligand. After activation of integrin, the β subunit extends and then the α subunit is exposed. The α subunit mainly mediates the reversible binding of integrin

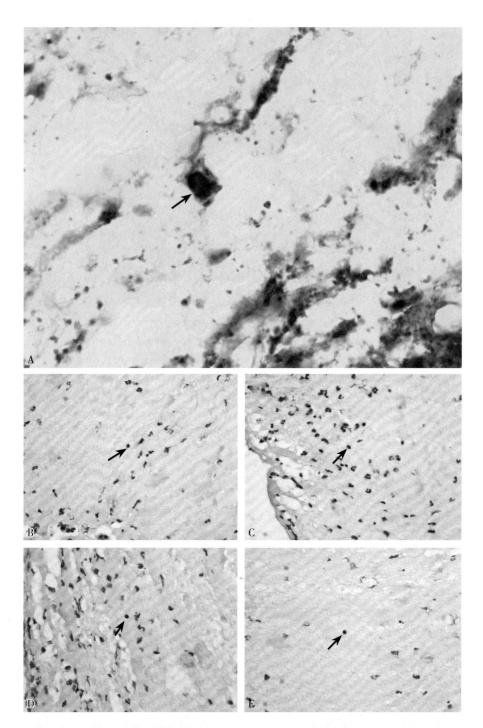

Figure 3-4-2. Immunohistochemistry of integrin β1 and its ligands. Arrow: dark-brown integrin β1 was expressed on the lymphocytes (A, ×1000). Expression of integrin β1 ligands (Laminin, B, ×400; Fibronectin, C, ×400; Collagen I, D, ×400; Collagen-II, Figure 2E, ×400) was not observed on the lymphocytes. (International Journal Of Clinical And Experimental Medicine,2014,7: 566-572)

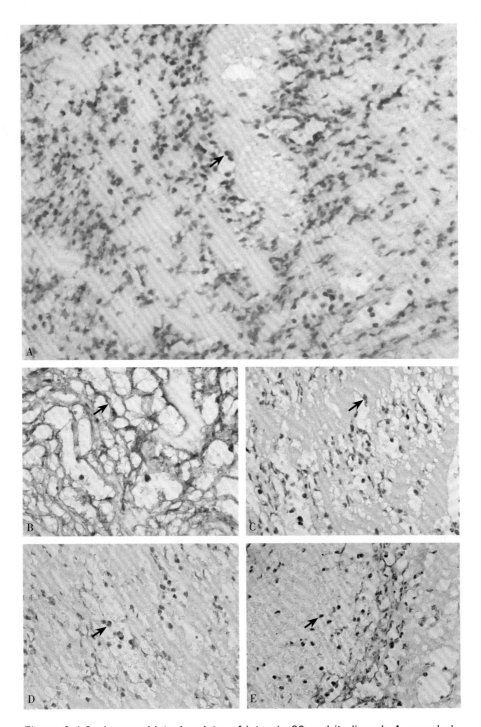

Figure 3-4-3   Immunohistochemistry of integrin β2 and its ligands.Arrow: dark-stained integrin β2 was expressed on the neutrophils (A, ×400) and bound fibrinogen (B, ×400). ICAM (C, ×400), factor X (D, ×400), and C3b (E, ×400) were expressed on neutrophils. (International Journal Of Clinical And Experimental Medicine,2014,7: 566-572)

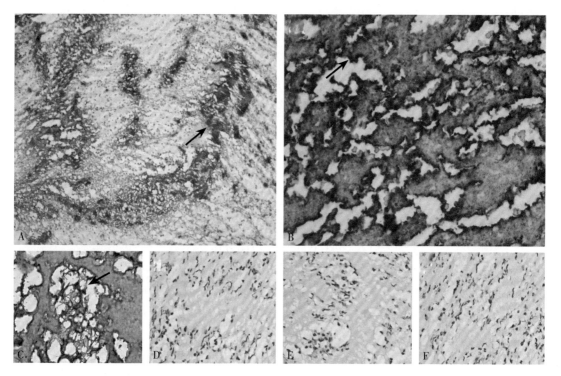

Figure 3-4-4. Immunohistochemistry of integrin β3 and its ligands.Arrow: dark-brown integrin β3 was expressed on platelets (A, ×200) and on the coral-like skeleton formed by platelets (B, ×400). Platelets and neutrophils bound fibrinogen to construct mesh-like structure (C, ×400). No expression of Fibronectin (D, ×400), Vitronectin (E, ×400) , vWF (F, ×400) was observed on these cells. (International Journal Of Clinical And Experimental Medicine,2014,7: 566-572)

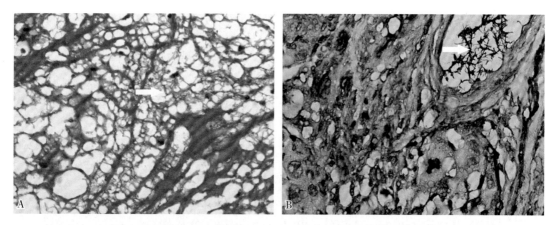

Figure 3-4-5   nest-like biological filter within the venous thrombus. Arrow: Mesh-like structure was nest-like biological filter (A, ×400, Masson staining), in which red blood cell dominant blood cells filled (C, ×400, Masson staining). In colon cancer, massive mesh-like structure (anti-fibrinogen antibody, 1 : 100, B, ×400) was observed in venules, and cancer cells were also observed in this mesh-like structure (anti-fibrinogen antibody, 1 : 100, D, ×400) (International Journal Of Clinical And Experimental Medicine,2014,7: 566-572)

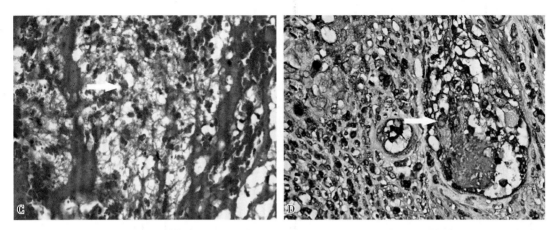

Figure 3-4-5(Continued)

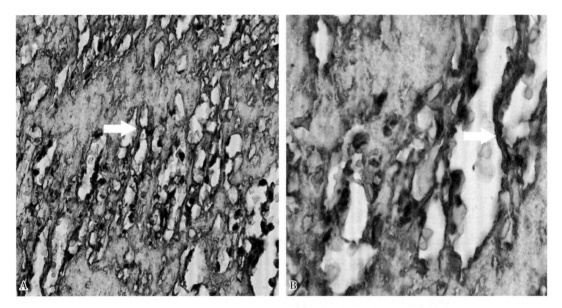

Figure 3-4-6   Factor Xa widely distributed on the surface of mesh-like structure. Arrow: dark-brown factor Xa was found on the surface of mesh-like structure (A, ×400; B, ×1000). This suggests factor Xa acts on the fibrinogen/fibrin (International Journal Of Clinical And Experimental Medicine,2014,7: 566-572)

to its ligand. The β subunit is responsible for signal transduction and regulation of integrin's affinity [3]. Integrin β1 is mainly expressed on lymphocytes [4], and its ligands include laminin, fibronetin, collagen, thrombospondin and VCAM-1 [5]. The binding of Integrin β1 and its ligands is involved in immune cell adherence, which can provide costimulation for activation of T cells. Integrin β2 is mainly expressed on the neutrophils and monocytes [6], and its ligands include fibrinogen, ICAM, factor X and C3b [7]. The binding of Integrin β2 and ligands is involved in immune cell adherence, inflammation and phagocytosis. Integrin β3 is expressed on the platelets [8] and its ligand includes fibrinogen, fibronetin, vitronectin, VWF and thrombospondin [9]. The binding of Integrin β3 and its ligands is involved in activation and aggregation of platelets.

Many cells are involved in inflammatory immune responses, including lymphocytes, neutrophiles and platelets. Light microscopy showed that the thrombi in acute pulmonary thromboembolism were red thrombi. Immunohistochemistry revealed that integrin β1 was distributed on lymphoctes. Laminin, fibronetin, collagen Ⅰ and Ⅱ, ligands of integrin β1, were not expressed on these cells. Integrin β2 was mainly distributed on neutrophils. The binding of activated integrin β2 with fibrinogen results in the formation of filamentous mesh. The ligands of integrin β2 (ICAM, factor X and C3b) were expressed on neutrophils, suggesting that the binding of integrin β2 with the ligands is involved in the thrombosis. Integrin β3 is distributed on platelets gathered in different shapes, which bind with fibrinogen to construct the filamentous mesh. No expression of fibronetin, vitronectin or vWF was observed on the platelets. The main protein component of acute venous thrombi is fibrinogen [1]. The result indicates the binding of platelet integrin β3 and neutrophil integrin β2 with ligand fibrinogen in thrombi is the early form of venous thrombosis.

In the thrombi, neutrophils and platelets are activated and bind to corresponding ligands, leading to inflammatory immune adhesion, which finally constructs filamentous mesh, a framework of venous thrombus. When the filamentous mesh is fully filled with red blood cell dominant blood cells, a red thrombus is formed. In the circulation, except for red blood cells, platelets and neutrophils have the largest amount. The binding of integrins on the membrane of platelets and neutrophils and their ligands is directly involved in the formation of acute venous thrombus. The binding of neutrophils and factor X can trigger the coagulation process and the activated factor X is converted to Xa and distributed on the fibrinogen, promoting soluble fibrinogenic thrombi to be transformed to fibrinic thrombi. Acute venous thrombosis is a main activation process of circulating neutrophils and platelets, and it is a whole process of integrin subunits β2 and β3 binding with their ligands, and a process of inflammatory immune adherence triggering coagulation reaction.

Thirty years ago, investigators developed and applied transient or permanent inferior vena cava filter in clinical practice to block the flow back of venous thrombi into the pulmonary artery, which may prevent the occurrence of PE [10]. In the study, the mesh-like structure in thrombi is similar to a biological filter, but what is the function of this mesh-like structure?

We have reported that virus-like microorganisms were observed in cytoplasm and intercellular substance of lymphocytes from peripheral venous blood of VTE patients with pulmonary hypertension and T cell immune dysfunction/disorder [11]. We also observed rod-shaped bacteria like microorganisms in apoptotic phagocytes from peripheral venous blood of patients with repeated PE/DVT and T cell immune dysfunction/disorder [12]. We also found DVT in the veins of multiple organs (such as pulmonary artery, kidney, liver and pancreas) of a patient who died of SARS [13]. These findings indicate that the onset of VTE has the involvement of infection of microorganisms. Moreover, the mRNA expression of T cells and NK cells was significantly down-regulated in patients with symptomatic VTE, as demonstrated by genomics data [14]. The amounts of CD_3, CD_8 and $CD_{16}CD_{56}$ T cells reduced significantly, the increased CD_4 level in patients with symptomatic VTE was consistent with findings in genomics [15]. The increased level of integrin subunit β1 in this study indicates the activation of lymphocytes, suggesting that the regulatory function of lymphocytes is enhanced. Malignancy is a disease related to immune dysfunction. Figures 3-4-5 B and D show that the mesh-like structure in the veins of cancer tissue is similar to that in venous thrombi. Furthermore, a variety of cancer cells were observed in this mesh like structure of veins in cancer tissue.

Acute venous thrombosis is an activation process of circulating lymphocytes, neutrophils and platelets, and it is a whole process of integrin subunit β1, β2 and β3 binding with their ligands, and a process of immune adherence, generating biological sieve and triggering coagulation reaction. Thus, we hypothesize that, when the infected cells or cancer cells can not be effectively and timely cleared in the presence of immune dysfunction/disorder, activated neutrophils and platelets bind to their ligands to construct biological filamentous mesh-like structure, which acts as a barrier to block the flow of infected cells or cancer cells. When the filamentous mesh-like structure was fully filled with red blood cell dominant blood cells, red venous thrombi occurred. The defensive biological filamentous mesh-like structure causes venous thrombosis.

(Published: Int J Clin Exp Med 2014;7(3):566-572.)

References

1. Wang L, Gong Z, Jiang J, Xu W, Duan Q, Liu J, et al. Confusion of wide thrombolytic time window for acute pulmonary embolism: mass spectrographic analysis for thrombus proteins. Am J Respir Crit Care Med. 2011; 184(1): 145-6.

2. Dorner M, Zucol F, Alessi D, Haerle SK, Bossart W, Weber M, Byland R, Bernasconi M, Berger C, Tugizov S, Speck RF, Nadal D. beta1 integrin expression increases susceptibility of memory B cells to Epstein-Barr virus infection. J Virol. 2010 Jul;84(13):6667-77.

3. van der Flier A, Sonnenberg A. Function and interactions of integrins. Cell Tissue Res. 2001; 305(3): 285-98.

4. Cavers M, Afzali B, Macey M, McCarthy DA, Irshad S, Brown KA. Differential expression of beta1 and beta2 integrins and L-selectin on CD_4 and CD_8 T lymphocytes in human blood: comparative analysis between isolated cells, whole blood samples and cryopreserved preparations. Clin Exp Immunol. 2002 Jan;127(1):60-5.

5. Fiorilli P, Partridge D, Staniszewska I, Wang JY, Grabacka M, So K, Marcinkiewicz C, Reiss K, Khalili K, Croul SE.

Integrins mediate adhesion of medulloblastoma cells to tenascin and activate pathways associated with survival and proliferation. Lab Invest. 2008 Nov;88(11):1143-56.

6. Rezzonico R, Chicheportiche R, Imbert V, Dayer JM. Engagement of CD11b and CD11c beta2 integrin by antibodies or soluble CD23 induces IL-1beta production on primary human monocytes through mitogen-activated protein kinase-dependent pathways. Blood. 2000;95(12):3868-77.

7. Schwarz M, Nordt T, Bode C, Peter K. The GP IIb/IIIa inhibitor abciximab (c7E3) inhibits the binding of various ligands to the leukocyte integrin Mac-1 (CD11b/CD18, alphaMbeta2). Thromb Res. 2002 Aug 15;107(3-4):121-8.

8. Fang J, Nurden P, North P, Nurden AT, Du LM, Valentin N, Wilcox DA. C560Rβ3 caused platelet integrin αII b β3 to bind fibrinogen continuously, but resulted in a severe bleeding syndrome and increased murine mortality. J Thromb Haemost. 2013 Jun;11(6):1163-71.

9. Coburn J, Magoun L, Bodary SC, Leong JM. Integrins alpha(v)beta3 and alpha5beta1 mediate attachment of lyme disease spirochetes to human cells. Infect Immun. 1998 ay;66(5):1946-52.

10. Athanasoulis CA, Kaufman JA, Halpern EF, Waltman AC, Geller SC, Fan CM.Inferior vena caval filters: review of a 26-year single-center clinical experience. Radiology. 2000 Jul;216(1):54-66.

11. Wang L, Gong Z, Liang A, et al. Compromised t-cell immunity and virus-like structure in a patient with pulmonary hypertension. Am J Respir Crit Care Med 2010; 182:434-5.

12. Wang L, Zhang X, Duan Q, Lv W, Gong Z, Xie Y, et al. Rod-like Bacteria and Recurrent Venous Thromboembolism. Am J Respir Crit Care Med. 2012; 186(7): 696.

13. Xiang-Hua Y, Le-Min W, Ai-Bin L, et al. Severe acute respiratory syndrome and venous thromboembolism in multiple organs. Am J Respir Crit Care Med 2010; 182:436-7.

14. Wang H, Duan Q, Wang L, Gong Z, Liang A, Wang Q, Song H, Yang F and Song Y. Analysis on the pathogenesis of symptomatic pulmonary embolism with human genomics. Int J Med Sci 2012; 9: 380-386.

15. Duan Q, Gong Z, Song H, Wang L, Yang F, Lv W, Song Y. Symptomatic venous thromboembolism is a disease related to infection and immune dysfunction. Int J Med Sci. 2012;9(6):453-61.

5. Nest-like biological venous filter within acute venous red thrombus

PE is an acute disease with high mortality and a sudden death rate of about 25% on autopsy [1]. To prevent the onset of PE, different kinds of filters such as nested vena cava filters were developed 30 years ago and had been applied in clinical practice to block DVT thrombi below the inferior vena cava reflowing to pulmonary artery.

In this study, several red thrombi were extracted via a 7F catheter from the pulmonary artery of a 50-year-old male with acute PE. Pathological sections were prepared and Masson staining was done. Light microscopy found spontaneous nest-like biological venous filter within the venous thrombus.

In the thrombus of acute PE, there distributes thrombus skeleton, which connects with filamentous grid to build a nest-like biological venous filter (Figure 3-5-1A), which is mainly filled with red blood cells (Figure 3-5-1B).

The sophisticated body always adjusts to the favorable direction of development and tends to balance stability and continuity between the internal and external environment. Biological venous filter is a result of the body's own regulation. What is the role? Manmade venous filter was used to block thrombus reflowing to pulmonary artery, what about the spontaneous nested biological venous filter within the thrombus blocking?

Smeeth et al. [2] have reported that acute infections were associated with an increased risk of VTE. We have reported that the functions of CD_3, CD_8, $CD_{16}CD_{56}$ and CD_{19} are compromised or disordered in more than 95% acute symptomatic VTE [3].

We reported that virus-like micro-organisms were detected under electron microscope in the cytoplasm of lymphocytes from the peripheral venous blood of VTE patients with pulmonary hypertension [4]. We also reported that electron microscopy showed rod-like bacteria in apoptotic phagocytic cells from the peripheral venous blood of a patient with recurrent PE/DVT [5]. We found biological venous filter formed in

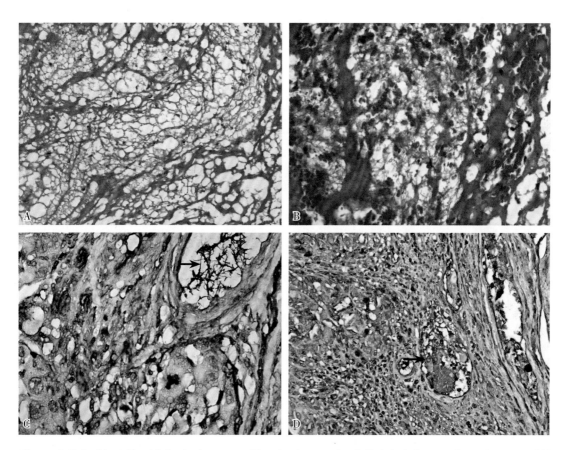

Figure 3-5-1　Nest-like biological venous filter is the result of fibrinic inflammation. In acute PE thrombus, there builds a nest-like biological venous filter (A, Masson×200), within which mainly filled with red blood cells(B, Masson×200); biological venous filter formed in veins surrounding cancer tissues(immunochemistry for fibrinogen, C×400, arrow); the filter was detained with cancer cells (immunochemistry for fibrinogen, D×400, arrow).

veins surrounding cancer tissues (Figure 3-5-1C), and the filter was detained with cancer cells (Figure 3-5-1D).

These results indicated that heterophilic antigens (pathogenic microorganisms or cancer cells) can not be timely or effectively cleared, so the biological venous filter becomes the protective screen. This protective screen is the local physical defense line of the body. When the filter is obstructed by blood cells and the blood flow is interrupted, venous red thrombus forms.

In the venous thrombus, there are irregular, coralliform thrombus skeleton and fibrous net, forming the nest-like biofilter (Figure 3-5-2,3-5-3). Thrombus skeleton is a product of platelet aggregation and the fibrous net is made of fibrinogen.

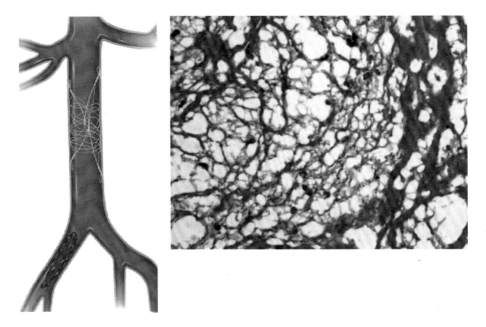

Figure 3-5-2   Shape of artificial nest-like inferior vena cava filter and venous biofilter. Left: Schema of artificial nest-like inferior vena cava filter; Right: nest-like structure of biofilter in the venous thrombus under a microscope. (International Journal Of Clinical And Experimental Medicine,2015,8(11):19804-19814)

The biological function of biofilter in the venous thrombus is still unclear. We have reported that there are cancer cells in this biofilter, suggesting that this biofilter may hinder the circulation of cancer cells and block the hematogenous metastasis of cancer cells. In addition, we also reported the virus-like microorganisms and rod-shaped bacteria in the lymphocytes and neutrophils, suggesting the presence of intracellular infection. The formation of intravenous biofilter means the existence of cells with intracellular infection / cancer cells and the loss of ability of immune cells to effectively clear foreign materials. The intravenous biofilter is a new barrier that

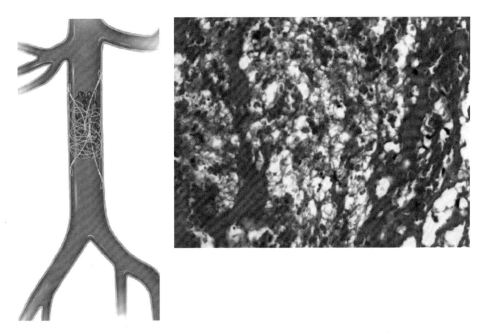

Figure 3-5-3   Artificial inferior vena cava filter blocks the back-flow of thrombus and blood cells in nest-like structure of biofilter. Left: Schema of artificial nest-like inferior vena cava filter. Back-flow of thrombus arrested in the artificial inferior vena cava filter; Right: under a microscope, erythrocyte-dominant blood cells were found in the nest-like structure of biofilter in the venous thrombus (International Journal Of Clinical And Experimental Medicine,2015,8(11):19804-19814)

spontaneously forms in the vein, indicating the re-construction of human defense system.

References

1. Lucena J, Rico A, Vázquez R, et al. Pulmonary embolism and sudden-unexpected death: prospective study on 2477 forensic autopsies performed at the Institute of Legal Medicine in Seville. J Forensic Leg Med. 2009;16(4):196-201.

2. Smeeth L, Cook C, Thomas S, et al. Risk of deep vein thrombosis and pulmonary embolism after acute infection in a community setting. Lancet 2006; 367:1075-9.

3. Duan Q, Gong Z, Song H, et al. Symptomatic Venous Thromboembolism Is a Disease Related to Infection and Immune Dysfunction Int J Med Sci. 2012; 9(6):453-461.

4. Wang L, Gong Z, Liang A, et al. Compromised t-cell immunity and virus-like structure in a patient with pulmonary hypertension. Am J Respir Crit Care Med, 2010, 182:434-435.

5. Lemin W, Xiaoyu Z, Qianglin D, Wei L, Zhu G, Yuan X, Aibin L, Yenan W. Rod-like Bacteria and Recurrent Venous Thromboembolism. Am J Respir Crit Care Med. 2012;186(7):696.

6. Venous Thrombosis is a product in proliferation of cancer cells

An 83 year old male received surgical intervention due to adenocarcinoma of the sigmoid colon. An 84-year old male underwent surgical intervention due to gastric cancer. HE staining and immunohistochemistry for fibrinogen (rabbit anti-human fibrinogen antibody [ab34269] abcam, 1 ∶ 100) were performed to observe the cancer cells and tissues (Figure 3-6-1, 3-6-2).

In the acute venous thrombus, the filamentous mesh-like structure formed by dark brown fibrinogens was identical to the filamentous mesh-like structure in the veins of cancers. This suggests that the pathogenesis of VTE in patients with cancer is related to the destruction of small veins and the intravenous formation of filamentous mesh-like

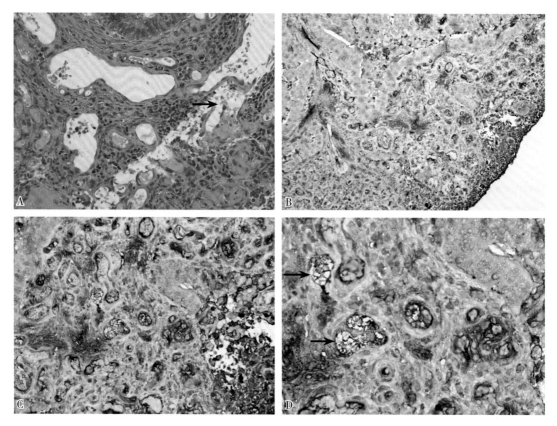

Figure 3-6-1   Pathology and immunohistochemistry of colon adenocarcinoma. A. Necrosis, granulation tissues, angiogenesis of capillaries and small veins in sigmoid colon adenocarcinoma; →disruption of small veins, and red blood cells and eosinophilic protein-like substances in venous vessels (HE,×200). B. Immunohistochemistry showed dark brown fibrinogens deposited in venous wall (×200). C. Dark brown fibrinogens deposited around cancer tissues (×200). D. →Dark brown fibrinogens in veins formed mesh-like structure (×400). (International Journal Of Clinical And Experimental Medicine,2014,7: 1319-1323)

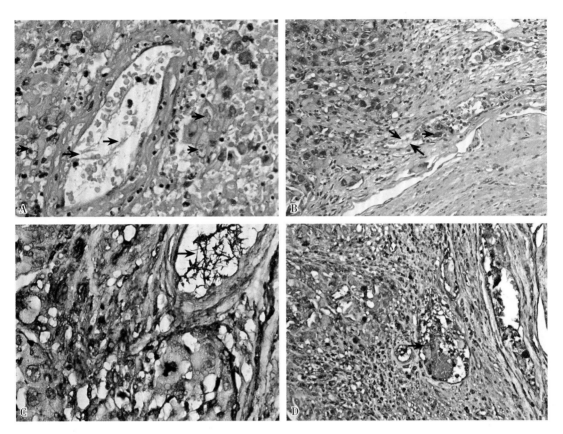

Figure 3-6-2   Pathology of colon adenocarcinoma showed hemorrhagic inflammation and fibrinic inflammation. A: Necrotic region in poorly differentiated gastric carcinoma presented with exudation of a large number of red blood cells. → red blood cells and eosinophilic filamentous protein-like substances in veins; →cancer cells with nuclear atypia surrounding veins (HE,×400); B. Dark brown fibrinogens in cancer tissues; →cancer embolus in veins (HE, ×200). C. filamentous mesh-like dark brown fibrinogens in veins of cancer tissues (×400); D. dark brown fibrinogens formed mesh-like structure which interfered with hematogenous metastasis of cancer cells (×200). (International Journal Of Clinical And Experimental Medicine,2014,7: 1319-1323)

structure by fibrinogen.

Our study showed the exudation of a large amount of red blood cells and a large amount of fibrinogens deposit in cancer tissues. These findings suggest that the cancer tissues damage the small veins and/or increase vascular permeability, which are characterized by hemorrhagic inflammation and fibrous inflammation. The small veins contain filamentous mesh-like structure formed by fibrinogens, in which cancer cells were found. This structure significantly interfered with the migration of cancer cells.

Fibrinogens convert to fibrins and deposit around cancer cells to form a barrier to block metastasis of cancer cells, which inhibit the migration of cancer cells. Electric microscopy and immunohistochemistry demonstrated the presence of fibrin in the primary cancer and metastatic cancer. These fibrins capsulated the primary cancer cells to inhibit the escape of cancer cells. In addition, these fibrinogens also formed stable skeleton in the extracellular matrix of cancer cells [1]. In the cancer, the intravenous fibrinogen formed mesh-like structure which becomes a barrier inhibiting the migration of cancer cells. The mesh-like structure not only inhibits the hematogenous metastasis of cancer cells but also blocks the back-flow of blood cells. The red blood cell dominant blood cells filling the mesh-like structure may cause VTE, which indicates the shift from defense to the opposite side. Our previous study showed that the main protein component of acute venous thrombi was fibrinogen [2]. Fibrinogens and fibrins constitute mesh-like structure, which becomes a nest-like filter in the veins. The blood cells stay in the filter forming red thrombi. The intravenous mesh-like structure in the cancer was consistent with the mesh-like structure in the venous red thrombi, as demonstrated by morphological examination and immunohistochemsitry.

The proliferation of cancer cells is usually faster than the growth of small blood vessels. Thus, the cancer is susceptible to ischemic necrosis, which is characterized by increase in vascular permeability and disruption of small blood vessels. The malignant tumor may invade the small blood vessels (mainly the small veins), which may also destroy the small vessels. Autopsy of patients with malignancies showed 50% of patients developed concomitant VTE [3]. We speculated that the prevalence of VTE in malignancy patients was higher than 50%. The morphological characteristics of proliferative cancer cells increase the risk for VTE in cancer patients, but the VTE may not be identified at early phases.

About 10-25% of VTE patients are diagnosed as malignancy within 2 years after diagnosis of VTE. Thus, patients with VTE of unknown cause might be a candidate of occult cancer with VTE as a first symptom [4]. This is of important significance for the diagnosis of cancer. On one hand, the cancerous VTE and non-cancerous VTE patients have obvious differences in the treatment, risk for VTE recurrence and survival time; on the other hand, malignant tumor may be diagnosed at an early phase due to the occurrence of VTE as an alarm, which promotes early diagnosis. On the basis of the above findings, the National Institute for Health and Clinical Excellence in England developed a CG144 guideline in 2012, which recommends the screening of malignant tumors in patients older than 40 years and with idiopathic VTE [4]. Roekshana regarded it as a milestone in the prevention and treatment of VTE [3].

Malignancy patients with concomitant VTE have identical nature in the occurrence of VTE to the occult cancer patients with VTE as an initial symptom. In these patients, VTE serves as a product in the proliferation of cancer cells and a result of focal fibrous inflammation after the disruption of small veins in cancers.

(Published: Int J Clin Exp Med 2014; 7: 1319-1323)

References

1. Hu L, Yang H, Su L, et al. Clinical research of the hypercoagulable state in 180 patients with malignant tumor. Med Res Edu 2010; 27(5): 30-32.

2. Wang L, Gong Z, Jiang J, Xu W, Duan Q, Liu J,Qin C. Confusion of wide thrombolytic time window for acute pulmonary embolism: mass spectrographic analysis for thrombus proteins. Am J Respir Crit Care Med. 2011;184:145-146.

3. Shaboodien R, Stansby G, Hunt BJ, Agarwal R. Unprovoked venous thromboembolism: assess for cancer. Lancet Oncol. 2012;13(10):973-4.

4. Chong LY, Fenu E, Stansby G, Hodgkinson S; Guideline Development Group. Management of venous thromboembolic diseases and the role of thrombophilia testing: summary of NICE guidance. BMJ. 2012;344:e3979.

Chapter 4

Cytological detection of core proteins

1. A New marker for diagnosis of VTE

In 2011, we reported that fibrinogen, rather than fibrin, was a major thrombus protein in acute PE [1]. The remaining proteins included serum albumin and cytoskeletal proteins. Fibrinogen makes embolus fragile, which theoretically explains the reason for wide thrombolytic time window: thrombolytic therapy can be extended to several days, 2 weeks, or even longer. It also explains why interventional fragmentation is effective for patients with acute PE.

The main component of red thrombus in acute VTE is fibrinogen. What is the relationship between fibrinogen and lymphocytes, leucocytes, platelets and erythrocytes? It is involved in the molecular mechanisms underlying the pathogenesis of acute VTE. Our pilot studies on the genomics, functional proteomics and informatics of acute VTE have demonstrated that the subunits of integrin β1, β2 and β3 are core proteins in the red thrombus [2]. The core proteins in thrombus bind to fibrinogen to generate unstable grid structure. When the grid structure is filled with erythrocytes, the soluble and fragile red thrombus forms. The subunits of integrin β1, β2 and β3 are distributed on the membranes of lymphocytes, leucocytes and platelets, respectively. As the configurations and expressions of these proteins change in VTE patients, the integrin subunits β1, β2 and β3 may serve as the early diagnostic markers of VTE. In the present study, 120 VTE patients diagnosed by imaging examinations and 120 sex and age matched non-VTE patients and healthy controls were recruited, and the expressions of integrin β1, β2 and β3 were detected in the peripheral blood cells.

Study population

A total of 120 inpatients with acute VTE were recruited from Apr 2011 to Dec 2012, including 47 males and 73 females, with an average age of 67.84±16.09 years (range: 24-90 years). All acute DVT patients were diagnosed by ultrasonography or selective intravenous angiography. Acute PE patients were diagnosed by CT pulmonary angiography (CTPA) or selective pneumoangiography. Patients with malignancies,

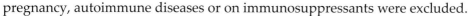

pregnancy, autoimmune diseases or on immunosuppressants were excluded.

During the same period, 120 sex and age matched non-VTE patients and healthy controls were also enrolled as controls. Non-VTE patients had no clinical symptoms of VTE and VTE was excluded by ultrasonography or CTPA. The study protocol was approved by the Ethics Committee of Tongji Hospital, and an informed consent was obtained from all patients in accordance with the declaration of Helsinki.

Blood collection and measurements

Detailed clinical history was collected immediately after patients were admitted to the hospital. A total of 2 ml of fasting peripheral blood samples were colleted from subjects in three groups and anti-coagulated with EDTA. Detection was carried out within two hours.

Monoclonal antibodies were employed in the detection of integrin $\beta1$(CD29), $\beta2$(CD18) and $\beta3$ (CD61) expression. Fluorescent antibodies against CD29, CD18 and CD61 were purchased from BD (USA). Briefly, 100 µl EDTA-anticoagulant peripheral blood was added into the test tubes and homotype control tubes were introduced simultaneously. According to different fluorescent markers, 20 µl of mouse IgG1-PC5, IgG1-FITC or IgG1-PE (mouse IgG2-PE substituted for IgG1-PE in the detection of CD29) was added. Subsequently, 20 µl of corresponding fluorescent antibodies were added. After mixing thoroughly, the mixture was kept in dark for 30 min at room temperature. Then, 500 µl of haemolysin (BECKMAN-COULTER, USA) was added into the tubes, followed by incubation at 37 ℃ for 30 min. After washing, 500 µl of sheath reagent was added to each tube, followed by flow cytometry (EPICS XL-4, BECKMAN-COULTER). A total of 10000 cells were analyzed in each detection. The percentage of positive cells was calculated, and results were analyzed by the built-in SYSTEM-II software.

Statistical analysis

Statistical analysis was performed with SPSS 18.0 software. According to the Kolmogorov-Smirnov analysis, the blood levels of integrins showed a skewed distribution. Thus, these variables were presented as medians (1st, 3rd quartiles). The medians and interquartile ranges were plotted in the figures as a box and whisker plot. In addition, differences in the variables between patients and controls were examined with Student's t-test or two-tailed Mann-Whitney U-test. The Chi-square test and Fisher's exact probabilities were employed for the comparison between observed and expected frequencies. Furthermore, the receiver operating characteristic (ROC) curves for predicting survival were plotted and analyzed to compare the diagnostic performance. Youden's index [3] was calculated, and the optimum diagnostic cutoff levels, sensitivity, specificity, positive and negative predictive values were analyzed according to the maximum of Youden's index. A value of P<0.05 was considered statistically significant.

Patients' characteristics

A total of 120 VTE patients and 120 non-VTE patients and healthy controls matched in age and sex were enrolled into this study. Among the 120 VTE patients, 72 (60.00%) were diagnosed with DVT and 48 (40.00%) with PE. There were 8 (6.67%) patients suffering from both DVT and PE. Patients' demographics, type of episodes, disease history and plasma integrin levels are shown in Table 4-1-1.

Table 4-1-1   The characteristics of VTE patients and non-VTE patients at baseline

Parameters	VTE Patients n=120	non-VTE Patients n=120	P
Demographics			
Age mean (SD)	67.84 (16.09)	68.20 (12.03)	0.845
Female (n, %)	73 (60.83%)	68 (56.67%)	0.600
Type of episode, n (%)			
DVT	72 (60.00%)		
PE	48 (40.00%)		
DVT + PE	8 (6.67%)		
Comorbidities (%)			
COPD	6(5.00%)	6 (5.00%)	1.000
CAD	35 (29.17%)	39(32.50%)	0.675
Diabetes mellitus	18 (15.00%)	16 (13.33%)	0.853
Hypertension	47 (39.17%)	40 (33.33%)	0.421
CI	19 (15.83%)	16 (13.33%)	0.715
Blood levels(pg/ml)			
Integrin $\beta 1$	14.50 (10.60,18.80)	7.85 (5.80,9.28)	0.000
Integrin $\beta 2$	94.90 (91.35,97.00)	88.95 (83.58, 91.48)	0.000
Integrin $\beta 3$	11.50 (9.77,15.65)	8.90(7.80, 10.40)	0.000

Blood integrin levels

Blood Integrin levels were quantified by flow cytometry. The median levels of integrin $\beta 1$, $\beta 2$ and $\beta 3$ were all significantly higher in VTE patients when comapred with non-VTE patients (P=0.000, 0.000 and 0.000, respectively) and healthy controls (P=0.000, 0.000 and 0.000, respectively). Between non-VTE patients and healthy controls, there was no statistical significance in the blood levels of integrin $\beta 1$, $\beta 2$ and $\beta 3$ (P=0.572, 0.544 and 0.547, respectively). (Figure 4-1-1)

ROC curve analysis

ROC curve analysis was utilized to assess diagnostic performance of these proteins.

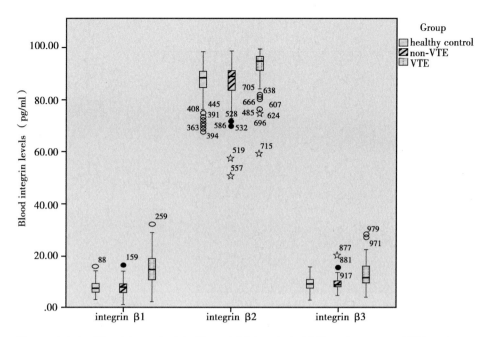

Figure 4-1-1   Blood integrin β1, β2 and β3 levels in VTE patients, non-VTE patients and healthy controls. Integrin levels were compared with Mann-Whitney U test. Significant differences in blood integrinβ1, β2 and β3 levels were observed between VTE patients and non-VTE patients (P=0.000, 0.000 and 0.000, respectively), and between VTE patients and healthy controls (P=0.000, 0.000, and 0.000, respectively). When compared between non-VTE patients and healthy controls, there were no significant differences(P=0.572, 0.544and 0.547, respectively). (International Journal Of Clinical And Experimental Medicine,2014,7: 2578-2584)

When a comparison was made between VTE patients and non-VTE patients, the AUC of integrin β1, integrin β2 and integrin β3 was 0.869 (P=0.000, 95%CI: 0.821-0.916), 0.809 (P=0.000, 95%CI: 0.752-0.867) and 0.742 (P=0.000, 95%CI: 0.676-0.809), respectively, and that of combined three integrins and D-Dimer was 0.917 (P=0.000, 95%CI: 0.878-0.956), and 0.811 (P=0.000, 95%CI: 0.754-0.868), respectively (Figure 4-1-2).

When a comparison was made between VTE patients and healthy controls, the AUC of integrin β1 integrin β2 and integrin β3 was 0.875 (P=0.000, 95%CI: 0.829-0.922), 0.828 (P=0.000, 95%CI: 0.774-0.882), and 0.721 (P=0.000, 95%CI: 0.655-0.786), respectively, and that of combined three integrins was 0.915 (P=0.000, 95%CI: 0.876-0.954) (Figure 4-1-3).

When a comparison was made between VTE patients and non-VTE patients plus healthy controls, the AUC of integrin β1, integrin β2 and integrin β3 was 0.870 (P=0.000, 95%CI: 0.825-0.915), 0.821 (P=0.000, 95%CI: 0.771-0.871) and 0.731 (P=0.000, 95%CI: 0.671-0.792), respectively, and that of combined three integrins was 0.916 (P=0.000, 95%CI: 0.878-0.953) (Figure 4-1-4).

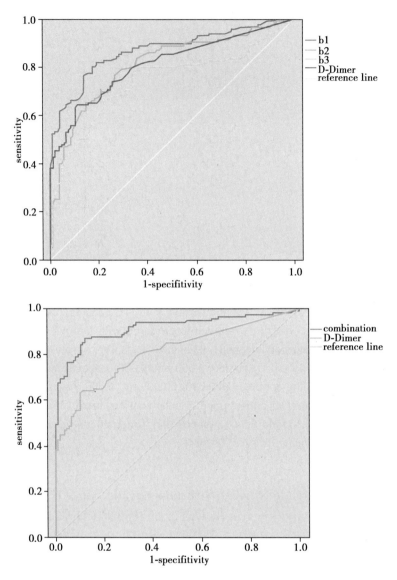

Figure 4-1-2   Receiver Operating Characteristic (ROC) curves for distinguishing VTE patients from non-VTE patients. The comparative ROC curves for all the three integrins (left), combination of three integrins(right) and D-Dimer are provided. The area under the curve (AUC) of integrin β1, integrin β2 and integrinβ3 was 0.869 (P=0.000, 95%CI: 0.821-0.916), 0.809 (P=0.000, 95%CI: 0.752-0.867) and 0.742 (P=0.000, 95%CI: 0.676-0.809), respectively, and that of combined three integrins and D-Dimer was 0.917 (P=0.000, 95%CI: 0.878-0.956), and 0.811 (P=0.000, 95%CI: 0.754-0.868), respectively. (International Journal Of Clinical And Experimental Medicine,2014,7: 2578-2584)

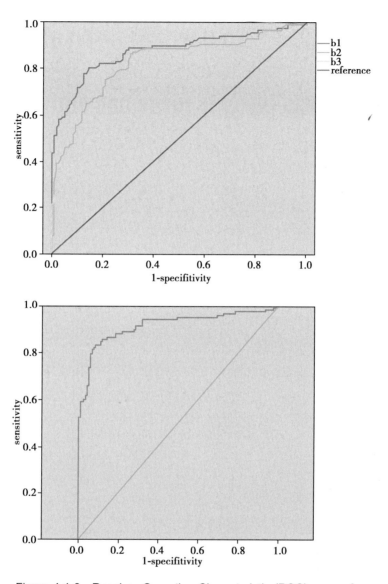

Figure 4-1-3   Receiver Operating Characteristic (ROC) curves for distinguishing VTE patients from healthy controls. The comparative ROC curves for all the three integrins (left) and the combination of integrins (right) are provided. The area under the curve (AUC) of integrin β1, integrin β2 and integrin β3 was 0.875 (P=0.000, 95%CI: 0.829-0.922), 0.828 (P=0.000, 95%CI: 0.774-0.882), and 0.721 (P=0.000, 95%CI: 0.655-0.786), respectively, and that of combined three integrins was 0.915 (P=0.000, 95%CI: 0.876-0.954). (International Journal Of Clinical And Experimental Medicine,2014,7: 2578-2584)

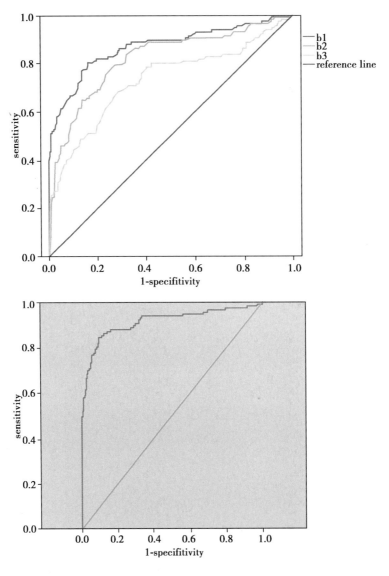

Figure 4-1-4   Receiver Operating Characteristic (ROC) curves for distinguishing VTE patients from non-VTE patients plus healthy controls. The comparative ROC curves for all the three integrins (left) and the combination of integrins (right) are provided. The area under the curve (AUC) was integrin β1, integrin β2 and integrin β3 was 0.870 (P=0.000, 95%CI: 0.825-0.915), 0.821 (P=0.000, 95%CI: 0.771-0.871) and 0.731 (P=0.000, 95%CI: 0.671-0.792), respectively, and that of combined three integrins was 0.916 (P=0.000, 95%CI: 0.878-0.953). (International Journal Of Clinical And Experimental Medicine,2014,7: 2578-2584)

Ages are shown as mean (SD), integrins as median (1st, 3rd quartiles), and categorical data as the number and percentage to the sample group. Age was compared with Student's t test. Gender was compared with chi-square test. Integrin level was compared with Mann-Whitney U test.

Abbreviations:DVT: deep venous thrombosis, PE: pulmonary embolism, COPD: chronic obstructive pulmonary disease, CAD: coronary artery disease, CI: cerebral infarction.

VTE patients usually have nonspecific clinical presentations, which are difficult to diagnose [4]. Recently a number of biomarkers have been evaluated with regard to their potential for predicting VTE, but results are currently contradictory among different labs [5-8]. In this study, we evaluated whether three integrins (β1, β2 and β3) could serve as promising biomarkers for VTE.

Integrins are transmembrane receptors that mediate the adhesion between cells and cells, and between cells and extracellular matrix (ECM). As signaling receptors, integrins play important roles in regulating the signaling pathways involved in the growth, proliferation, differentiation, and migration of cells. Integrins are heterodimeric glycoproteins. In humans, there are 20 different integrins with special ligands formed by specific non-covalent binding of 18 α and 9 β subunits [9].

The subunit of β1 integrin is mainly expressed on the membranes of lymphocytes and platelets. The corresponding ligands are laminin, collagen, thrombospondin, fibronetin and vascular cell adhesion molecule 1 (VCAM-1) [10]. The subunit of β2 integrin is mainly expressed on the membranes of neutrophils and monocytes, and the corresponding ligands are fibrinogen, intercellular adhesion molecule (ICAM), factor X, and ic3b [11]. The β3 subunit of integrin is expressed on the membrane of platelet and the corresponding ligands are fibrinogen, fibronetin, vitronectin, vWF, thrombospondin and so on [12].

The results of our pilot study showed that the β1, β2 and β3 subunits of integrin were core proteins of red thrombus in VTE. Through binding of these core proteins to ligands, platelets aggregate to the coralloid structures, and then core proteins bind to fibrinogen to generate grid structures of the thrombus. It is basic mechanism underlying the pathogenesis of VTE.

The present study showed that the blood levels of integrins β1, β2, and β3 were all significantly higher in VTE patients than in non-VTE patients and healthy controls. The ROC curves showed that the AUC of integrin β1, β2 and β3 subunits in diagnosing acute VTE was 0.870, 0.821 and 0.731, respectively. When integrins β1, β2, and β3 were combined as a diagnostic marker for VTE, the AUC was 0.916, and the sensitivity, specificity, positive and negative predictive value were 84.6%, 90.8%, 81.7% and 92.0%, respectively, which indicates the potential for using blood integrins β1, β2, and β3 as biomarkers for the diagnosis of VTE (Table 4-1-2).

Table 4-1-2 Diagnostic performance of three integrins for VTE

	Integrinβ1	Integrinβ2	Integrin β3	β1+β2+β3
AUC	0.870	0.821	0.731	0.916
Optimum cutoff (pg/ml)	10.29	91.10	10.35	
sensitivity	80.3%	78.6%	68.4%	84.6%
specificity	83.7%	73.7%	71.2%	90.8%
Positive predictive value	71.1%	59.4%	54.3%	81.7%
negative predictive value	89.3%	87.6%	81.8%	92.0%

D-Dimer is a degradation product of cross-linked fibrin and forms immediately when the thrombin-generated fibrin clots are degraded by the plasmin. Thus, it reflects the whole activation of blood coagulation and fibrinolysis. Being the best-recognized biomarker for initial assessment of suspected VTE, D-Dimer with a negative value may safely rule out both DVT and PE with a sensitivity of 83%-96% and a negative predictive value of nearly 100%. However, because of its poor specificity of about 43%-71% in diagnosing VTE [13-17], D-Dimer testing has to be included in comprehensive sequential diagnostic strategies that incorporate clinical probability assessment and imaging techniques. Our study showed that combined measurement of thrombus core proteins (different integrin subunits) had a moderate sensitivity (84.6%), but a high specificity (90.8%) in diagnosing VTE. In patients, especially those with elevated D-Dimer, measurement of integrins is useful in the diagnosis of VTE and can avoid excessive imaging examinations.

According to the treatment time, anticoagulant therapies in VTE can be grouped into three classes: 1 month, 3 months and lifelong anticoagulant therapy. Hemorrhage is an important complication of anticoagulation therapy. There is lack of objective indicators for determining the course of warfarin therapy and deciding the reduction or withdrawal of warfarin therapy [18-22]. In this study, during 6-12 month follow-up, no evidence of VTE recurrence was found in 10 VTE patients whose integrin subunits β1, β2, and β3 restored to the normal range after Warfarin withdrawal. These findings suggest that when the expressions and configurations of integrin subunits β1, β2, and β3 return to the normal levels, they no longer bind to the corresponding ligands. Thus, the thrombosis was destroyed gradually. These may be potential indicators to determining the duration of oral anticoagulant therapy.

(Published:Int J Clin Exp Med 2014; 7: 2578-2584.)

References

1. Wang L, Gong Z, Jiang J, et al. Confusion of wide thrombolytic time window for acute pulmonary embolism: mass spectrographic analysis for thrombus proteins. Am J Respir Crit Care Med 2011; 184:145-146.

2. Xie Y, Duan Q, Wang L, et al. Genomic characteristics of adhesion molecules in patients with symptomatic pulmonary embolism. Mol Med Rep 2012; 6:585-590.

3. Youden WJ (1950) Index for rating diagnostic tests. Cancer 3: 32-35.

4. Torbicki A, Perrier A, Konstantinides S, et al. Guidelines on the diagnosis and management of acute pulmonary embolism: the Task Force for the Diagnosis and Management of Acute Pulmonary Embolism of the European Society of Cardiology (ESC) Eur Heart J. 2008;29:2276-2315.

5. Righini M, Perrier A, De Moerloose P, Bounameaux H. D-Dimer for venous thromboembolism diagnosis: 20 years later. J Thromb Haemost. 2008;6:1059 -1071.

6. Di Nisio M, Squizzato A, Rutjes AW, Buller HR, Zwinderman AH, Bossuyt PM. Diagnostic accuracy of D-dimer test for exclusion of venous thromboembolism: a systematic review. J Thromb Haemost. 2007;5:296 -304.

7. Rectenwald JE, Myers DD Jr, Hawley AE, Longo C, Henke PK, Guire KE, Schmaier AH, Wakefield TW. D-dimer, P-selectin, and microparticles: novel markers to predict deep venous thrombosis. A pilot study. Thromb Haemost. 2005; 94:1312-1317.

8. Ingrid Pabinger and Cihan Ay. Biomarkers and Venous Thromboembolism. Arterioscler Thromb Vasc Biol. 2009;29:332-336.

9. Vyas SP, Vaidya B. Targeted delivery of thrombolytic agents: role of integrin receptors. Expert Opin Drug Deliv. 2009; 6(5):499-508.

10. Lityńska A, Przybylo M, Ksiazek D, et al. Differences of alpha3beta1 integrin glycans from different human bladder cell lines. Acta Biochim Pol 2000; 47(2):427-34.

11. Solovjov DA, Pluskota E, Plow EF. Distinct roles for the alpha and beta subunits in the functions of integrin alphaMbeta2. J Biol Chem 2005; 280(2):1336-45. Epub 2004 Oct

12. Gerber DJ, Pereira P, Huang SY, et al. Expression of alpha v and beta 3 -integrin chains on murine lymphocytes. ProcNatl Acad Sci USA. 1996; 93(25):14698-703.

13. Bounameaux H, Cirafici P, Schneider PA et al. Measurement of D-dimer in plasma as diagnostic aid insuspected pulmonary embolism. Lancet 337:196-200; 1991.

14. Bozic, M, Blinc A, Stegnar M. D-dimer, other markers of haemostasisactivation and soluble adhesion molecules in patients with different clinicalprobabilities of deep vein thrombosis. Thromb Res 108:107-114; 2002.

15. Declerck PJ, Mombaerts P, Holvoet P et al. Fibrinolyticresponse and fibrin fragment D-dimer levels in patients with deep veinthrombosis. Thromb. Haemostasis 58:1024-1029; 1987.

16. Di Nisio, M.; Squizzato, A.; Rutjes, A. W.;et al.Diagnostic accuracy of D-dimer test for exclusion of venousthromboembolism: a systematic review. J. Thromb. Haemostasis 5: 296-304; 2007.

17. Di Nisio M, Squizzato A, Rutjes AWS, et al. Diagnostic accuracy of D-dimer test for exclusion ofvenous thromboembolism: a systematic review. J Thromb Haemost 2007; 5(2): 296- 304.

18. Kahn SR, Lim W, Dunn AS, et al. Prevention of VTE in nonsurgical patients: Antithrombotic Therapy and Prevention of Thrombosis, 9th ed: American College of Chest Physicians Evidence-Based Clinical Practice Guidelines. Chest. 2012; 141(2 Suppl):e195S-226S.

19. Le Gal G, Kovacs MJ, Carrier M, et al. Validation of a diagnostic approach to exclude recurrent venous thromboembolism. J Thromb Haemost 2009; 7: 752-59.

20. Palareti G, Cosmi B, Legnani C, et al. D-dimer testing to determine the duration of anticoagulation therapy. N Engl J Med 2006; 355: 1780-89.

21. Prandoni P, Lensing AW, Prins MH, et al. Residual venous thrombosis as a predictive factor of recurrent venous thromboembolism. Ann Intern Med 2002; 137: 955-60.

22. Bounameaux H, Righini M. Thrombosis: duration of anticoagulation after VTE: guided by ultrasound? Nat Rev Cardiol 2009; 6: 499-500.

2. Increased expressions of integrin subunits β1, β2 and β3 in patients with acute infection

American College of Chest Physicians, ACCP, has put forward various risk factors of acquired VTE, including surgery, trauma, infection, tumor, aging, pregnancy, long-bedding and immobilization, etc [1]. Acute infection is commonly faced in clinical practice, and there is a 2-3 times increased incidence of VTE in patients with community-acquired or hospital-acquired infections [2-4].

Acute venous thrombosis is red thrombus, which is composed of red blood cells, platelets, white blood cells and plasma proteins. In 2011, we reported that the main component of red thrombus in acute PE patients was fibrinogen, rather than fibrin, with only a small quantity of cellular cytoskeletal and plasma proteins [5]. Fibrinogenic thrombus is dissolvable, which can explain why delayed thrombolytic therapy is effective for acute and subacute VTE and thrombi are autolytic in some VTE patients. However, the action mechanism of fibrinogen in thrombosis remains unclear. We hypothesized that, due to the binding of fibrinogens (ligands) and activated receptors on surfaces of various leukocytes, platelets and lymphocytes, the thrombus protein network is constructed and red thrombus forms, with erythrocytes and plasma components filled in the spaces. In our previous studies [6, 7], genomics analysis, proteomics analysis and bioinformatics analysis of acute venous thrombi of PE patients confirmed that integrins β1, β2 and β3 were the core proteins of acute venous thrombi. Integrin β1 is mainly localized on lymphocytes, integrin β2 is mainly localized on neutrophils and integrin β3 is mainly localized on platelets. Moreover, activated integrin β3 was involved in the accumulation of platelets, receptors of integrin β2 and β3 bound to fibrinogens to form the biofilter-like grid structure of thrombi filled with red blood cells, forming red thrombi.

Acute infection is a risk factor of VTE, but why is acute infection prone to VTE?

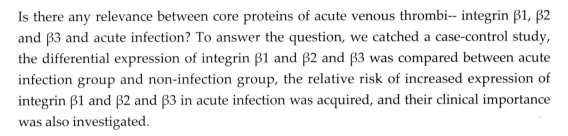

Is there any relevance between core proteins of acute venous thrombi-- integrin β1, β2 and β3 and acute infection? To answer the question, we catched a case-control study, the differential expression of integrin β1 and β2 and β3 was compared between acute infection group and non-infection group, the relative risk of increased expression of integrin β1 and β2 and β3 in acute infection was acquired, and their clinical importance was also investigated.

Study population

A total of 230 patients with acute infection diagnosed from April 2011 to April 2012 in the emergency unit were recruited into this study, including 118 males and 112 females, aged 23-93 years, with a mean age of 72.53 years old. The classification of acute infection was according to the previously reported criteria [8], and the patients included 197 cases of respiratory tract infections (pneumonia and bronchitis), 19 cases of urinary tract infection, 19 cases of skin and soft tissue infection, 7 cases of abdominal infection (liver and gallbladder and gastrointestinal tract) and 8 cases of sepsis without clear foci. Among them, 18 cases were complicated with two kinds of infections. All infected patients were diagnosed in our hospital. Meanwhile, 230 age and gender matched inpatients without infection served as the control group, including 114 males and 116 females, aged 21-98 years (mean 70.31 years). Patients with cancer, autoimmune disease or patients taking immunosuppressive drugs were excluded. Patients with clinical symptomatic thrombus were also excluded. This study was approved by the Ethics Committee of Affiliated Tongji Hospital of Tongji University, and informed consent was obtained before study.

Blood collection and measurements

Detailed clinical data were collected from each acute infection patient and control patient on admission. Blood routine test, hsCRP and d-dimer were detected. HsCRP was detected by immune scatter turbidimetry, using Siemens BNII specific protein and auxiliary reagent. D-dimer was detected by Latex enhanced immune turbidimetric turbidity method, using SYSMEX CA1500 automatic blood coagulation analyzer. Fasting venous blood (2 ml) was collected from the cubital vein in the morning and anti-coagulated with EDTA. Two hours later, the anti-coagulated blood was processed as follows.

Monoclonal antibodies against integrin β1 (CD29), β2 (CD18) and β3 (CD61) (BD company) were used to detect the integrin β1, β2 and β3, respectively. Three tag monoclonal antibodies (BECKMAN-COULTER) were used for CD_3, CD_4 and CD_8 detection. In brief, 100 μl of EDTA treated blood was added to each tube and control tube was also included. Then, 20 μl of mouse IgG1-PC5, IgG1-FITC or IgG1-PE was added (20 μl of IgG2-PE was mixed with CD29), followed by addition of corresponding fluorescence antibodies (20 μl). Following vortexing, incubation was done in dark for 30 min at room temperature. Then, 500 μl of hemolysin (BECKMAN-COULTER) was added, followed by incubation at 37°C for 30 min. Following washing, 500 μl of sheath fluid was added to each tube, followed by flow cytometry (EPICS XL-4; BECKMAN-COULTER). The PMT voltage, fluorescence compensation and sensitivity of standard fluorescent microspheres (EPICS XL-4; BECKMAN-COULTER) were used to adjust the flow cytometer and a total of 10000 cells were counted for each tube. The corres ponding cell population in the scatterplot of isotype controls was used to set the gate, and the proportion of positive cells was determined in each quadrant (%). SYSTEM-II was used to process the data obtained after flow cytometry.

Statistical analysis

SPSS18.0 statistical software was used for statistical analysis. Normality test was performed for all measurement data using the Kolmogorov-Smirnov test, with P> 0.05 as normal distribution. Data of normal distribution were expressed as means ± SD and were compared with t test between groups. Corrected t-test was applied when heterogeneity of variance. Non-normal data were expressed as median P_{50} and interquartile range (P_{25}-P_{75}), and group comparison was analyzed using nonparametric test (Mann-Whitney U test). Measurement data were compared using chi-square test. The association degree between two categorical variables was analyzed by calculating the relative risk (Relative Risk, RR). P <0.05 was considered statistically significant for all tests.

Patients' characteristics

A total of 230 patients with acute infection and 230 patients without acute infection matched in age and sex were enrolled into this study. Among the 230 patients with acute infection, 197(85.7%) were diagnosed with respiratory tract infections (RTI), 19(8.3%) were diagnosed with urinary tract infection (UTI), 19(8.3%) were diagnosed with skin infection, 7(3.0%) were diagnosed with intra-abdominal infection and 8(3.5%) were diagnosed with septicaemia. Patients' demographics, type of infection and comorbidities are shown in Table 4-2-1.

Table 4-2-1   The baseline characteristics of 230 patients with acute infection and controls

	Acute infection(%) N=230	Controls(%) N=230	P value
Mean age(SD)	72.53(16.81)	70.31(12.61)	0.110
Gender, male	118(51.3)	114(49.6)	0.780
Acute infection			
Respiratory tract infection(RTI)	197(85.7)		
Urinary tract infection(UTI)	19(8.3)		

	Acute infection(%) N=230	Controls(%) N=230	P value
Skin infection	19(8.3)		
Intra-abdominal infection	7(3.0)		
septicaemia	8(3.5)		
Comorbidities			
CAD	104(51.2)	114(49.6)	0.349
Hypertension	102(44.3)	84(41.4)	0.106
CI	63(27.4)	53(23.0)	0.284
DM	48(20.9)	42(18.3)	0.557
COPD	34(14.8)	22(9.6)	0.116

Ages are shown with mean (SD); categorical data are shown with the number and percentage of the sample group.Ages were compared by Student's t test.The frequency of categorical data was compared with the chi-square test. Abbreviations:CAD, coronary artery disease; CI, cerebrovascular infarction; DM, diabetes mellitus; COPD, chronic obstructive pulmonary disease.

Plasma D-Dimer and HsCRP levels

The median levels of D-Dimer and HsCRP were all significantly higher in patients with acute infection when compared with patients without acute infection (P=0.000 and 0.000) (Table4-2-2).

Table 4-2-2　Expression of cellular immunity, HsCRP and d-dimer in patients with acute infection and controls

	Acute infection(pg/ml) N=230	controls(pg/ml) N=230	P value
CD_3	63.46(12.28)	64.93(12.40)	0.203
CD_4	36.82(11.55)	37.29(10.96)	0.654
CD_8	23.02(9.01)	22.16(8.11)	0.287
CD_4CD_8	1.80(1.10-2.70)	1.80(1.40-2.70)	0.376
$CD_{16}CD_{56}$	14.95(9.18-20.68)	9.90(5.48-17.20)	0.008
CD_{19}	7.8(4.20-11.33)	10.1(6.33-15.23)	0.018
D-Dimer	0.28(0.11-0.49)	0.09(0.05-0.25)	0.000
HsCRP	28.85(10.70-55.80)	3.10(0.98-14.70)	0.000

CD_3, CD_4, CD_8 were shown with mean (SD) and compared by Student's t test.CD_4/CD_8,$CD_{16}CD_{56}$,CD_{19},D-Dimer and HsCRP were shown with median(p25th-p75th)and compared by Mann-Whitney U test.

Blood cellular immunity related variables

When comparing cellular immunity related variables (CD_3, CD_4, CD_8, CD_4/CD_8, $CD_{16}CD_{56}$ and CD_{19}), we found significant differences of $CD_{16}CD_{56}$ and CD_{19} (P=0.008, P=0.018) between the two groups. $CD_{16}CD_{56}$ was markedly increased in acute infection patients, while CD_{19} was reduced (see Table 4-2-2).

Blood integrin levels

Compared with the control group, the expression of integrin β1, β2 and β3 was markedly increased in the acute infection group (P=0.000, 0.002 and 0.001, respectively) (Table 4-2-3). The relative risk ratio (RR) of increased integrin β1, β2 and β3 in acute infection patients was 1.424 (95%CI: 1.156-1.755, P=0.001), 1.535, (95%CI: 1.263-1.865, P=0.000) and 1.20 (95%CI: 0.947-1.521, P=0.148), respectively (Table 4-2-3, 4).

Table 4-2-3 Expression of integrin β1, β2 and β3 in patients with acute infection and controls. integrinβ1, β2, β3 were shown with mean(SD) and compared by Student's t test

	Acute infection (pg/ml) N=230	Controls (pg/ml) N=230	P value
Integrin β1	11.82(6.10)	9.63(4.62)	0.000
Integrin β2	91.05(7.28)	88.94(6.99)	0.002
Integrin β3	10.37(4.05)	9.29(3.05)	0.001

Combined integrin β1, β2 and β3 analysis (integrin β1, β2 and β3 increased at the same time means rise, otherwise normal) showed the relative risk ratio (RR) of increase in acute infection patients was 2.962 (95%CI: 1.621-5.410, P=0.001) (see Table 4-2-4).

Table 4-2-4 Relative risk of increased expression of integrin β1, β2 and β3 in acute infection

	Acute infection above/normal	Controls above/normal	RR	95%CI	P value
integrinβ1	120/108	85/145	1.424	1.156-1.755	0.001
integrinβ2	133/90	89/140	1.535	1.263-1.865	0.000
integrinβ3	94/134	79/151	1.20	0.947-1.521	0.148
Combination of integrinβ1,β2 and β3	38/189	13/217	2.962	1.621-5.410	0.000

Acute infection is a risk factor of thrombotic diseases [9-12]. In 2006, Smeeth et al. reported [2] that the risk for DVT was increased by 1.91 folds within 2 weeks to 6 months after acute respiratory tract infection. Similar finding is also noted in patients after urinary infection. Recently, in two large case-control studies [3,4], results also demonstrate that acute infection increases the risk for VTE by 2~3 folds after adjustment of other risk factors of VTE, and this risk is the highest within 2 weeks after acute infection.

Our results showed that the expression of integrins β1, β2 and β3 was markedly increased in patients with acute infection. The risk for increased integrin β1, β2 and β3 expression in patients with acute infection was respectively 1.424, 1.535 and 1.20 folds higher than that in patients without acute infection. Combined integrin β1, β2 and β3 analysis showed that the relative risk for patients with acute infection was 2.962 folds higher than that in patients without acute infection. These results may explain the increased risk of VTE in acute infection patients. For patients with acute infection and increased integrin β1, β2 and β3, early treatment and prevention should be given, in order to reduce the incidence of VTE in high-risk groups.

Integrins are cell adhesion receptors, and they play an important role in the interaction between cells and extracellular matrix (ECM), and cell-cell interactions [13]. Integrins are heterodimers consisting of noncovalently linked α and β transmembrane glycoprotein subunits. They consist of at least 18 α and 8 β subunits, producing 24 different heterodimers [14]. The α and β subunits separate from each other once the integrin is activated, and then the α subunit binds the ligand. The β1 subunit is expressed mainly on cell surface of lymphocytes, and its ligands consist of laminins, collagens, thrombospondin, vascular cell adhesion molecule 1 and fibronectin [14,15]. The β2 subunit is distributed on cell surface of neutrophils and monocytes, and ligands for this subunit include fibrinogen, complement component iC3b, intracellular adhesion molecule-1, factor X and so on [16,17]. The β3 subunit is observed on platelets, and this subunit binds fibrinogen, fibronectin, vitronectin von Willebrand factor (vWF) and thrombospondin [18,19]. At rest, the integrin receptor does not bind to corresponding ligand. When the α subunit is separated from the β subunit, the integrin is activated. The α subunit mainly mediates the reversible binding of receptor to corresponding ligand. The β subunit is responsible for the signal transduction and the regulation of integrin affinity [20-22].

In addition, our results revealed that the acute infection patients had a tendency toward disordered cellular immunity. Our previous studies [23,24] also showed that the VTE patients had compromised cellular immunity. These findings suggest that acute infection patients with compromised cellular immunity have an increased risk for VTE. A weakened immune system could be the basic condition of VTE occurrence. When the immune system can not timely and effectively remove intravenous antigens of heterotypic cells, the platelets and white blood cells will be activated and bound to fibrinogens to form the biofilter-like grid structure of thrombi, which are filled with red blood cells, forming red thrombi. The disease process was from the body's defense to venous thrombosis.

(Published: *International Journal of Medical Sciences* 2015; 12(8): 639-643)

References

1. Kahn SR1, Lim W, Dunn AS, Cushman M, Dentali F, Akl EA, Cook DJ, Balekian AA, Klein RC, Le H, Schulman S, Murad MH. Prevention of VTE in nonsurgical patients: Antithrombotic Therapy and Prevention of Thrombosis, 9th ed: American College of Chest Physicians Evidence-Based Clinical Practice Guidelines. Chest. 2012;141(2 Suppl):e195S-226S.

2. Smeeth L, Cook C, Thomas S, Hall AJ, Hubbard R, Vallance P. Risk of deep vein thrombosis and pulmonary embolism after acute infection in a community setting. Lancet 2006; 367:1075-9.

3. Clayton TC, Gaskin M, Meade TW. Recent respiratory infection and risk of venous thromboembolism: case-control study through a general practice database. Int J Epidemiol 2011; 40:819-27.

4. Schmidt M, Horvath-Puho E, Thomsen RW, Smeeth L, Sørensen HT. Acute infections and venous thromboembolism. J Intern Med. 2011 Oct 25. doi: 10.1111/j.1365 -2796. 2011. 02473.x. [Epub ahead of print]

5. Wang L, Gong Z, Jiang J, Xu W, Duan Q, Liu J,Qin C. Confusion of wide thrombolytic time window for acute pulmonary embolism: mass spectrographic analysis for thrombus proteins. Am J Respir Crit Care Med. 2011;184:145-146.

6. Xie Y, Duan Q, Wang L, Gong Z, Wang Q, Song H, Wang H. Genomic characteristics of adhesion molecules in patients with symptomatic pulmonary embolism. Mol Med Rep 2012; 6:585-590.

7. Wang LM, Duan QL, Yang F, Yi XH, Zeng Y, Tian HY, Lv W, Jin Y. Activation of circulated immune cells and inflammatory immune adherence are involved in the whole process of acute venous thrombosis Int J Clin Exp Med 2014;7(3):566-572.

8. Smeeth L, Thomas SL, Hall AJ, Hubbard R, Farrington P, Vallance P. Risk of myocardial infarction and stroke after acute infection or vaccination. N Eng J Med 2004;351:2611-8.

9. Meier CR, Jick SS, Derby LE, Vasilakis C, Jick H. Acute respiratory-tract infections and risk of first-time acute myocardial infarction. Lancet 1998;351:1467-71.

10. Clayton TC, Capps NE, Stephens NG, Wedzicha JA,Meade TW. Recent respiratory infection and the risk of myocardial infarction. Heart 2005;91:1601-2.

11. Clayton TC, Thompson M, Meade TW. Recent respiratory infection and risk of cardiovascular disease: case-control study through a general practice database. Eur Heart J2008;29:96-103.

12. Warren-Gash C, Smeeth L, Hayward AC. Influenza as a trigger for acute myocardial infarction or death from cardiovascular disease: a systematic review. Lancet Infect Dis 2009;9:601-10.

13. Barczyk M, Carracedo S and Gullberg D. Integrins. Cell Tissue Res 2010; 339: 269-280.

14. Cavers M, Afzali B, Macey M, McCarthy DA, Irshad S and Brown KA. Differential expression of beta1 and beta2 integrins and L-selectin on CD_4 and CD_8 T lymphocytes in human blood: comparative analysis between isolated cells, whole blood samples and cryopreserved preparations. Clin Exp Immunol 2002; 127: 60-65.

15. Fiorilli P, Partridge D, Staniszewska I, Wang JY, Grabacka M, So K, Marcinkiewicz C, Reiss K, Khalili K and Croul SE. Integrins mediate adhesion of medulloblastoma cells to tenascin and activate pathways associated with survival

and proliferation. Lab Invest 2008; 88: 1143-1156.

16. Rezzonico R, Chicheportiche R, Imbert V and Dayer JM. Engagement of CD11b and CD11c beta2 integrin by antibodies or soluble CD23 induces IL-1beta production on primary human monocytes through mitogen-activated protein kinase-dependent pathways. Blood 2000; 95: 3868-3877.

17. Schwarz M, Nordt T, Bode C and Peter K. The GP IIb/IIIa inhibitor abciximab (c7E3) inhibits the binding of various ligands to the leukocyte integrin Mac-1 (CD11b/CD18, alphaMbeta2). Thromb Res 2002; 107: 121-128.

18. Fang J, Nurden P, North P, Nurden AT, Du LM, Valentin N and Wilcox DA. C560Rbeta3 caused platelet integrin alphaII b beta3 to bind fibrinogen continuously, but resulted in a severe bleeding syndrome and increased murine mortality. J Thromb Haemost 2013; 11: 1163-1171.

19. Coburn J, Magoun L, Bodary SC and Leong JM. Integrins alpha(v)beta3 and alpha5beta1 mediate attachment of lyme disease spirochetes to human cells. Infect Immun 1998; 66: 1946-1952.

20. Takada Y, Ye X, Simon S. The integrins. Genome Biol. 2007;8(5):215.

21. Xiong JP, Stehle T, Diefenbach B, Zhang R, Dunker R, Scott DL, Joaachimiak A, Goodman SL, Arnaout MA. Crystal structure of the extracellular segment of integrin alpha Vbeta3. Science. 2001 Oct 12; 294(5541):339-45.

22. Humphries MJ. Integrin structure. Biochem Soc Trans. 2000;28(4):311-39.

23. Lemin Wang, Haoming Song, Zhu Gong, Qianglin Duan, Aibin Liang. Acute pulmonary embolism and dysfunction of CD_3CD_8 T cell immunity. Am J Respir. Crit. Care Med.2011;Dec 184:1315.

24. Haoming Song, Lemin Wang, Zhu Gong, Aibin Liang, Yuan Xie, Wei Lv, Jinfa Jiang, Wenjun Xu, Yuqin Shen.T cell-meiated immune deficiency or compromise in patients with CTEPH. Am J Respir Crit. Care Med.2011;183(3):417-8.

3. Increased expressions of integrin subunits β1, β2 and β3 in patients with cancer

Cancer is one of the most common risk factors of VTE. The incidence of VTE in patients with cancer is about 4%~20%, and it has been a leading cause of death in cancer patients [1-3]. There is evidence showing that about 20% clinical first-episode patients with idiopathic VTE have been diagnosed malignant tumor in 6 months to 2 years. The prevalence of VTE in patients with malignancy is 4-7 times higher than that of patients without malignancy [4,5]. VTE has been an important contributor to morbidity and mortality among patients with cancer [6]. Why do malignancy patients have a high incidence of VTE? The molecular mechanisms are not clear. Acute venous thrombosis is red thrombus, which is composed of red blood cells, platelets, white blood cells and plasma proteins. In 2011, we reported that the main component of red thrombus in acute PE patients was fibrinogen, rather than fibrin, with only a small quantity of cellular cytoskeletal and plasma proteins [7]. In our further studies, genomics, proteomics and bioinformatics analyses of acute venous thrombi of PE patients confirmed that integrins β1, β2 and β3 were the core proteins of acute venous thrombi [8,9]. Integrin β1 is mainly localized on lymphocytes, integrin β2 is mainly localized on neutrophils and integrin β3 is mainly localized on platelets. Moreover, activated integrin β3 is involved in the accumulation of platelets and the receptors of integrins β2 and β3 are bound to fibrinogens to form the biofilter-like grid structure of thrombi, which are filled with red blood cells to form red thrombi. We also found that the filamentous mesh-like structure was widespread in the veins of cancers, and a large amount of red blood cells and cancer cells were found in this biofilter-like grid structure [10]. Integrin β1, β2, β3 subunits are core proteins and potential biomarkers of VTE [11]. Is there any relevance between core proteins of acute venous thrombi-integrin β1, β2 and β3 and cancer? In this study we will explore the expression of Integrin β1, β2, β3 subunits in patients with cancer and investigate their clinical importance.

Study population

A total of 144 inpatients with cancer diagnosed from April 2011 to April 2012 in the affiliated Tongji Hospital of Tongji University were recruited into this study, including 90 males and 54 females, aged 25-91 years, with a mean age of 67.36 years old. Cancers included lung cancer, intestinal cancer, hepatic cancer, gastric cancer, prostate cancer, breast cancer, esophageal cancer, pancreatic cancer, cervical cancer, kidney cancer, ovarian cancer, bladder cancer, nasopharyngeal cancer and laryngeal cancer. All cancers were confirmed by imaging or pathology. Meanwhile, 200 cases of age and gender matched inpatients without cancer were recruited as the control group, including 114 males and 86 females, aged 21-93 years (mean 68.17 years). Cancer was excluded in the control group by clinical symptoms, signs and imaging. Patients with acute infection, autoimmune disease or patients taking immunosuppressive drugs were excluded. Patients with clinical symptomatic venous thrombus were also excluded. This study was approved by the Ethics Committee of Affiliated Tongji Hospital of Tongji University, and informed consent was obtained before study.

Blood collection and measurements

Detailed clinical data were collected from each cancer patient and control patient on admission. Blood routine test, hsCRP and d-dimer were detected. HsCRP was detected by immune scatter turbidimetry, using Siemens BNII specific protein and auxiliary reagent. D-dimer was detected by Latex enhanced immune turbidimetric turbidity method, using SYSMEX CA1500 automatic blood coagulation analyzer. Fasting venous blood (2 ml) was collected from the cubital vein in the morning and anti-coagulated with EDTA. Two hours later, the anti-coagulated blood was processed as follows.

Monoclonal antibodies against integrin β1 (CD29), β2 (CD18) and β3 (CD61) (BD company) were used to detect the integrins β1, β2 and β3, respectively. Three tag monoclonal antibodies (BECKMAN-COULTER) were used for detection of CD_3, CD_4 and PC5, FITC, and PE label were used for CD_8, CD_3, CD_4 and CD_8, respectively. $CD_{16}CD_{56}$

and CD_{19} also used PE label. In brief, 100 μL of EDTA treated blood was added to each tube and control tube was also included. Then, 20 μL of mouse IgG1-PC5, IgG1-FITC or IgG1-PE was added (20 μL of IgG2-PE was mixed with CD29), followed by addition of corresponding fluorescence antibodies (20 μL). Following vortexing, incubation was done in dark for 30 min at room temperature. Then, 500 μL of hemolysin (BECKMAN-COULTER) was added, followed by incubation at 37°C for 30 min. Following washing, 500 μL of sheath fluid was added to each tube, followed by flow cytometry (EPICS XL-4; BECKMAN- COULTER). The PMT voltage, fluorescence compensation and sensitivity of standard fluorescent microspheres (EPICS XL-4; BECKMAN-COULTER) were used to adjust the flow cytometer and a total of 10000 cells were counted for each tube. The corresponding cell population in the scatterplot of isotype controls was used to set the gate, and the proportion of positive cells was determined in each quadrant (%). SYSTEM-II was used to process the data obtained after flow cytometry.

Statistical analysis

SPSS18.0 statistical software was used for statistical analysis. Normality test was performed for all measurement data using the Kolmogorov-Smirnov test, with P>0.05 as normal distribution. Data of normal distribution were expressed as means ± SD and were compared with student's t-test between groups. Corrected t-test was applied when heterogeneity of variance. Non-normal data were expressed as median P_{50} and interquartile range (P_{25}-P_{75}), and group comparison was analyzed using nonparametric test (Mann-Whitney U test). Measurement data were compared using chi-square test. The association degree between two categorical variables was analyzed by calculating the relative risk (Relative Risk, RR). P<0.05 was considered statistically significant for all tests.

Patients' characteristics

A total of 144 patients with cancer and 200 patients without cancer matched in age and sex were enrolled into this study. The 144 cancer patients included, 43 (29.86%) lung cancer, 25 (17.73%) intestinal cancer, 17 (12.06) hepatic cancer, 13 (9.22%) gastric cancer, 11 (7.8%) prostate cancer, 10 (7.09%) breast cancer, 6 (4.26%) esophageal cancer, 6 (4.26%) pancreatic cancer, 3 (2.13%) cervical cancer, 2 (1.42%) kidney cancer, 2 (1.42%) ovarian cancer, 2 (1.42%) bladder cancer, 2 (1.42%) nasopharyngeal cancer and 2 (1.42%) laryngeal cancer. Patients' demographics, type of cancer and comorbidities are shown in Table 4-3-1. The median levels of D-Dimer and HsCRP were all significantly higher in patients with cancer when compared with patients without cancer (P=0.000 and 0.000). In comparisons of the cellular immunity related variables (CD_3, CD_4, CD_8, CD_4/CD_8, $CD_{16}CD_{56}$ and CD_{19}), significant differences were found between the two groups: CD_3, CD_4, CD_4/CD_8 and CD_{19} were markedly decreased in patients with cancer

Table 4-3-1   The baseline characteristics of 144 patients with cancer and controls

	Patients with cancer (%) N=144	Controls (%) N=200	P value
Mean age (SD)	67.36 (12.67)	68.17 (12.09)	0.549
Gender, male	90 (62.5)	114 (57.0)	0.319
Cancer typing			
Lung cancer	43 (29.86)		
Intestinal cancer	25 (17.73)		
Hepatic cancer	17 (12.06)		
Gastric cancer	13 (9.22)		
Prostate cancer	11 (7.8)		
Breast cancer	10 (7.09)		
Esophageal cancer	6 (4.26)		
Pancreatic cancer	6 (4.26)		
Cervical cancer	3 (2.13)		
Kidney cancer	2 (1.42)		
Ovarian cancer	2 (1.42)		
Bladder cancer	2 (1.42)		
Nasopharyngeal cancer	2 (1.42)		
Laryngeal cancer	2 (1.42)		
Comorbidities			
CAD	15 (10.42)	30 (15)	0.199
Hypertension	34 (23.61)	51 (25.5)	0.705
CI	18 (12.5)	37 (18.5)	0.140
DM	29 (20.14)	36 (18)	0.676

Ages are shown with mean (SD); categorical data are shown with the number and percentage of the sample group. Ages were compared by Student's t test. The frequency of categorical data was compared with the chi-square test. Abbreviations: CAD, coronary artery disease; CI, cerebrovascular infarction; DM, diabetes mellitus.

(P=0.004, P=0.000, P=0.000 and P=0.000 respectively), while CD_8 and $CD_{16}CD_{56}$ were increased (P=0.000 and P=0.035) (Table 4-3-2). When compared with the control group, the expression of integrins β1 and β3 were markedly increased in patients with cancer (P=0.000 and P=0.008), while integrin β2 was only mildly increased in patients with cancer (P=0.274) (Table 4-3-3). The relative risk ratios (RR) of increased integrins β1, β2 and β3 in patients with cancer were 1.655 (95% CI: 1.321-2.074, P=0.000), 1.314, (95% CI: 1.052-1.642, P=0.021) and 1.852 (95% CI: 1.097-3.126, P=0.028), respectively. Combined integrin β1, β2 and β3 analysis showed (integrin β1, β2 and β3 increased at the same time means rise, otherwise normal) the relative risk ratio (RR) of increase in patients with cancer was 4.895 (95% CI: 1.645-14.563, P=0.002) (Table 4-3-4).

Table 4-3-2　Expression of cellular immunity, HsCRP and d-dimer in patients with cancer and controls

	Patients with cancer (pg/ml) N=144	Controls (pg/ml) N=200	P value
CD$_3$	60.71 (14.64)	64.91 (12.29)	0.004
CD$_4$	32.31 (11.30)	37.35 (11.26)	0.000
CD$_8$	25.00 (9.77)	22.16 (7.94)	0.005
CD$_4$CD$_8$	1.30 (0.87-2.08)	1.80 (1.40-2.50)	0.000
CD$_{16}$CD$_{56}$	11.95 (9.92-16.18)	9.75 (5.43-15.75)	0.035
CD$_{19}$	6.64 (3.88-12.10)	10.20 (6.35-15.28)	0.000
D-Dimer	0.19 (0.05-0.39)	0.08 (0.05-0.24)	0.000
HsCRP	11.40 (4.70-44.05)	3.00 (0.83-14.90)	0.000

CD$_3$, CD$_4$, CD$_8$ were shown with mean (SD) and compared by Student's t test. CD$_4$/CD$_8$, CD$_{16}$CD$_{56}$, CD$_{19}$, D-Dimer and HsCRP were expressed as median (p25th-p75th) and compared by Mann-Whitney U test.

Table 4-3-3　Expression of integrin β1, β2 and β3 in patients with cancer and controls

	Patients with cancer (pg/ml) N=144	Controls (pg/ml) N=200	P value
Integrin β1	12.34 (5.40)	9.63 (4.53)	0.000
Integrin β2	89.82 (6.63)	88.99 (7.12)	0.274
Integrin β3	10.33 (3.55)	9.39 (2.99)	0.008

integrinβ1, β2, β3 were shown with mean (SD) and compared by Student's t test.

Table 4-3-4　Relative risk of increased expression of integrin β1, β2 and β3 in patients with cancer

	Patients with cancer above/normal	Controls above/normal	RR	95% CI	P value
integrinβ1	87/57	73/127	1.655	1.321-2.074	0.000
integrinβ2	78/65	83/117	1.314	1.052-1.642	0.021
integrinβ3	28/116	21/179	1.852	1.097-3.126	0.028
Combination of integrinβ1, β2 and β3	14/129	4/196	4.895	1.645-14.563	0.002

Integrins are a kind of widespread cell surface receptors, which mediate interactions between cells and cells, and between cells and extracellular matrix (ECM). As signal receptors, integrins play an important role in the cell growth, migration, proliferation and differentiation of many aspects, and are one of the key members of the family of cell adhesion molecules [12]. Integrins are heterodimers consisting of noncovalently linked α and β transmembrane glycoprotein subunits. They consist of at least 18 α and 8 β subunits, producing 24 different heterodimers [13]. The β1 subunit is expressed mainly on cell surface of lymphocytes, and its ligands consist of laminins, collagens, thrombospondin, vascular cell adhesion molecule 1 and fibronectin [14]. The β2 subunit is distributed on cell surface of neutrophils and monocytes, and ligands for this subunit include fibrinogen, complement component iC3b, intracellular adhesion molecule-1, factor X and so on [15]. The β3 subunit is observed on platelets, and this subunit binds fibrinogen, fibronectin, vitronectin von Willebrand factor (vWF) and thrombospondin [16].

Cancer is a risk factor of VTE, and VTE is an important cause of death in cancer [17-19]. This study explored the expression of integrin β1, β2, β3 subunits in patients with cancer, the results showed that integrin β1, β2, β3 subunits were all increased in patients with cancer, among which integrin subunits β1 and β3 were increased significantly. The relative risk ratios (RR) of increased integrins β1, β2 and β3 in patients with cancer were 1.655, 1.314 and 1.852 respectively. Combined integrin β1, β2 and β3 analysis showed that the relative risk ratio (RR) of increase in patients with cancer was 4.895. As core proteins of venous thrombosis, the increased expression of integrins β1, β2 and β3 in patients with cancer may explain the relatively high risk of VTE in cancer patients.

The plasma levels of hsCRP and d-dimer were all significantly higher in patients with cancer in this study. As nonspecific inflammation markers, hsCRP was associated with venous thrombosis [20]. Elevated levels of serum hsCRP are a risk factor of VTE in cancer patients, which shows the role of nonspecific inflammation in the prone of VTE in patients with cancer [21]. Our study has shown that the incidence of VTE in patients with malignant tumor is the result of nonspecific inflammatory repair of small veins after being destroyed by tumor cells invasion, as demonstrated by morphological examination and immunohistochemistry [10]. This is different from infective inflammation. D-dimer is a degradation product of cross-linked fibrin that is formed immediately after thrombin-generated fibrin clots are degraded by plasmin and reflects a global activation of blood coagulation and fibrinolysis. Being the best-recognized biomarker for the initial assessment of suspected VTE, d-dimer has a high sensitivity of 83%-96%, but a poor specificity (around 40%) [22-24]. As core proteins of venous thrombosis, integrins β1, β2 and β3 have been proven to be a new useful biomarker of VTE both with a high sensitivity and an approving specificity in our previous study [11]. For patients with cancer who have increased integrins β1, β2 and β3, early treatment and prevention should be given in order to reduce the incidence of VTE in high-risk groups.

In this study, the cellular immune function was reduced or disordered in patients with cancer. Our previous studies had shown that VTE patients had association with compromised cellular immunity [25,26]. A weakened immune system could be the basic condition of VTE occurrence. These findings suggest that malignant tumor patients with compromised cellular immunity possess the intrinsic basic conditions for VTE and thus have an increased risk for VTE.

　　(published: Int J Clin Exp Med 2015;8(2):2772-2777)

References

1. Chew HK, Wun T, Harvey D, Zhou H, White RH. Incidence of venous thromboembolism and its effect on survival among patients with common cancers. Arch Intern Med 2006; 166: 458-64.

2. Khorana AA, Liebman HA, White RH, Wun T, Lyman GH. The risk of venous thromboembolism in patients with cancer. American Society of Clinical Oncology. Cancer Thromb; 2008. pp. 240-8.

3. Chew HK, Wun T, Harvey DJ, Zhou H, White RH. Incidence of venous thromboembolism and the impact on survival in breast cancer patients. J Clin Oncol 2007; 25: 70-6.

4. Wun T, White RH. Epidemiology of cancer-related venous throm-boembolism. Best Pract Res Clin Haematol 2009; 22: 9-23.

5. Blom JW, Doggen CJ, Osanto S, Rosendaal FR. Malignancies, pro-thrombotic mutations, and the risk of venous thrombosis. JAMA 2005; 293: 715-22.

6. Lyman GH, Khorana AA, Falanga A, Clarke-Pearson D, Flowers C, Jahanzeb M, Kakkar A, Kuderer NM, Levine MN, Liebman H, Mendelson D, Raskob G, Somerfield MR, Thodiyil P, Trent D, Francis CW; American Society of Clinical Oncology. American Society of Clinical Oncology Guideline:recommendations for venous throm- boembolism prophylax is and treatment in patients with cancer.J Clin Oncol 2007; 25: 5490-5505.

7. Wang L, Gong Z, Jiang J, Xu W, Duan Q, Liu J, Qin C. Confusion of wide thrombolytic time window for acute pulmonary embolism: mass spectrographic analysis for thrombus proteins. Am J Respir Crit Care Med 2011; 184: 145-146.

8. Xie Y, Duan Q, Wang L, Gong Z, Wang Q, Song H, Wang H. Genomic characteristics of adhesion molecules in patients with symptomatic pulmonary embolism. Mol Med Rep 2012; 6: 585-590.

9. Wang LM, Duan QL, Yang F, Yi XH, Zeng Y, Tian HY, Lv W, Jin Y. Activation of circulated immune cells and inflammatory immune adherence are involved in the whole process of acute venous thrombosis Int J Clin Exp Med 2014; 7: 566-572.

10. Le-Min Wang, Qiang-Lin Duan, Xiang-Hua Yi, Yu Zeng, Zhu Gong, Fan Yang. Venous thromboembolism is a product in proliferation of cancer cells. Int J Clin Exp Med 2014; 7: 1319-1323.

11. Yanli Song , Fan Yang, Lemin Wang, Qianglin Duan, Yun Jin, Zhu Gong. Increased expressions of integrin subunit $\beta1$, $\beta2$ and $\beta3$ in patients with venous thromboembolism: new markers for venous thromboembolism. Int J Clin Exp Med 2014; 7: 2578-2584.

12. Barczyk M, Carracedo S and Gullberg D. Integrins. Cell Tissue Res 2010; 339: 269-280.

13. Cavers M, Afzali B, Macey M, McCarthy DA, Irshad S and Brown KA. Differential expression of beta1 and beta2 integrins and L-selectin on CD_4 and CD_8 T lymphocytes in human blood: comparative analysis between isolated cells, whole blood samples and cryopreserved preparations. Clin Exp Immunol 2002; 127: 60-65.

14. Lityńska A, Przybylo M, Ksiazek D, Laidler P. Differences of alpha3beta1 integrin glycans from different human

bladder cell lines. Acta Biochim Pol 2000; 47: 427-34.

15. Solovjov DA, Pluskota E, Plow EF. Distinct roles for the alpha and beta subunits in the functions of integrin alphaMbeta2. J Biol Chem 2005; 280: 1336-45.

16. Gerber DJ, Pereira P, Huang SY, Pelletier C, Tonegawa S. Expression of alpha v and beta 3 16-integrin chains on murine lymphocytes. Proc Natl Acad Sci USA 1996; 93: 14698-703.

17. Sorensen HT, Mellemkjaer L, Olsen JH, Baron JA. Prognosis of cancers associated with venous thromboembolism. N Engl J Med 2000; 343: 1846-50.

18. Prandoni P, Falanga A, Piccioli A. Cancer and venous thromboembolism. Lancet Oncology 2005; 6: 401-10.

19. Khorana AA, Francis CW, Culakova E, Kuderer NM, Lyman GH. Thromboembolism is a leading cause of death in cancer patients receiving outpatient chemotherapy. J Thromb Haemost 2007; 5: 632-4.

20. Vormittag R, Vukovich T, Schönauer V, Lehr S, Minar E, Bialonczyk C, Hirschl M, Pabinger I. Basal high-sensitivity-C-reactive protein levels in patients with spontaneous venous thromboembolism. Thrombosis and Haemostasis. 2005; 93: 488-93.

21. Kröger K, Weiland D, Ose C, Neumann N, Weiss S, Hirsch C, Urbanski K, Seeber S, Scheulen ME. Risk factors for venous thromboembolic events in cancer patients. Annals of Oncology 2006; 17: 297-303.

22. Bounameaux H, Cirafici P, de Moerloose P, Schneider PA, Slosman D, Reber G, Unger PF. Measurement of D-dimer in plasma as diagnostic aid in suspected pulmonary embolism. Lancet 1991; 337: 196-200.

23. Bozic M, Blinc A, Stegnar M. D-dimer, other markers of haemostasis activation and soluble adhesion molecules in patients with different clinical probabilities of deep vein thrombosis. Thromb Res 2002; 108: 107-114.

24. Di Nisio M, Squizzato A, Rutjes AW, Büller HR, Zwinderman AH, Bossuyt PM. Diagnostic accuracy of D-dimer test for exclusion of venous thromboembolism: a systematic review. J Thromb Haemost 2007; 5: 296-304.

25. Haoming S, Lemin W, Zhu G, Aibin L, Yuan X, Wei L, Jinfa J, Wenjun X, Yuqin S. T cell-mediated immune deficiency or compromise in CTEPH patients. Am J Respir Crit Care Med 2011; 183: 417-8.

26. Wang L, Song H, Gong Z, Duan Q, Liang A. Acute Pulmonary Embolism and Dysfunction of CD_3 CD_8 T Cell Immunity. Am J Respir Crit Care Med 2011; 184: 1315.

4. Expression of the same or different proteins in venous thromboembolism and different risk factor group patients

In this study, we report that there was expression of specific proteins in patients with symptomatic VTE, and the expression of these proteins was compared between VTE group patients and those with different risk factor groups (acute infection, malignancy, autoimmune diseases, trauma /surgery). In addition, the role of these proteins in the risk for VTE was assessed.

Subjects and Methods

The subjects included patients with a definite diagnosis between March, 2011, and Feb, 2012, in Tongji Hospital of Tongji University. Patients were grouped by specific diseases based on the national standards by professionals, and the results were analyzed by

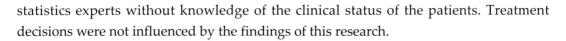

statistics experts without knowledge of the clinical status of the patients. Treatment decisions were not influenced by the findings of this research.

Patients and controls

A total of 1006 subjects (male=53%; female=47%; mean age=67.40±16.26) were enrolled from Departments of Cardiology, Internal Emergency, Oncology, Rheumatology, and Surgical Emergency of Shanghai Tongji Hospital, and divided into six groups.

The VTE group (within 3 months of onset, n=72) consisted of patients with DVT and/or PE, and the diagnosis was confirmed by imaging, and the patients received anticoagulant therapy with low molecular heparin or warfarin orally.

The acute infection group (n=330) included patients with infections of respiratory tract (pneumonia or bronchitis, n=168), urinary tract (n= 54), skin, soft-tissue (n= 25), intra-abdominal (gastrointestinal or hepatobiliary infections) (n=64), or sepsis (no site identified) (n= 19). The patients received anti-infection and comprehensive therapy.

The malignancy group (clinical stage III-IV, n=144) included lung cancer (n=56), gastric cancer (n=23), esophagus cancer (n=12), rectum cancer (n=14), pancreatic cancer (n=4), hepatic cancer (n=9), breast cancer (n=18), and brain cancer (n=8). A total of 47 cancer patients received chemotherapy, and the others received comprehensive therapy including chemotherapy, radiotherapy, immunization therapy and treatment by Chinese herbs.

The autoimmune diseases group (mild to moderate, n=103) included rheumatoid arthritis (n=39), systemic lupus erythematosus (n=32), Sjogren's syndrome (n=17), and connective tissue disease (n=15). They all received conventional immunoregulation and/ or Chinese medicine treatments. The trauma /surgery group (n=111) included 79 cases of several trauma (multiple injuries, n=36; head injury, n=28; traumatic fractures, n=15) and 32 surgical patients (cervical or lumbar vertebra surgery, n=16; gastric cancer surgery, n=5; intestinal cancer surgery, n=11) under general or local anesthesia for more than 30 min. The control group (non-risk factor group) included patients with atherosclerotic heart disease or/and hypertension (n=246), but without clinically symptomic VTE, and patients with acute infection, cancer, autoimmune diseases, trauma or recent surgical treatment were excluded.

Methods for detection

1) Levels of integrins β1, β2 and β3 in all individuals were detected and analyzed by EPICS XL-4 flow cytometry (Beckman-Coulter) using System II software. Fluorescent antibodies were provided by BD Company.

2) Patients were placed in a sitting position, and peripheral blood (2 ml) was collected from the median cubital vein and anti-coagulated with EDTA. After mixing, flow cytometry was done within 2 h.

3) 100 μl EDTA was added to each tube for anti-coagulation. Isotype control was also included. Integrin β1 and integrin β2 were mixed with 20 μl mouse IgG1-PE, and integrin β3 was mixed with 20 μl mouse IgG2-PE. Then, 20 μl fluorescent antibody was added to the above solution. After misce bene, incubation was done at room temperature in dark for 30 min. After addition of 500 μl hemolysin, incubation was done at 37℃ for 30 min. Following washing, 500 μl sheath fluid was added and then detected by flow cytometry.

The standardized BECKMAN-COULTER fluorescent microspheres were used to adjust the PMT voltage, fluorescence compensation, sensitivity, and the detection protocol was determined. A total of 10000 cells were collected in each tube. The scattered plot of isotype control was used for gating at corresponding cells. Integrin β1 and integrin β2 gating were lymphocytes, and integrin β3 gating was platelets. According to the fluorescence intensity in each quadrant, the proportion of positive cells was calculated (%). Data were analyzed with SYSTEM-II software.

Statistical analysis

Continuous variables were expressed as means ± SD or medians (interquartile range), and categorical variables were expressed as frequencies (percentages). Control ranges of integrin positive cells were determined from control individuals. The control ranges of integrins β1 and β3 positive cells were calculated as the mean ± 2SD, and were 3.14 to 13.90% and 4.39 to 14.7%, respectively (Table 4-4-1). Using the 5th-95th percentiles, we determined control range of integrins β2 positivity (non-normally distributed) of 73.40 to 95.30 (see Table 4-4-1). Integrin levels above the upper limit of the control range were considered positive, while levels below the upper limit of the control range were considered negative (see Table 4-4-1).

A total of 1006 inpatients were divided into: symptomatic VTE group, acute infection group, malignancy group, autoimmune diseases group, trauma /surgery group and control group. Expression of integrins was detected in these groups.

Compared with control group, the integrin β1 expression in VTE group and subjects with different risk factors (acute infection, malignancy and autoimmune diseases) increased markedly (P<0.001, <0.01). However, compared with control group, the integrin β1 expression in trauma /surgery group was not significantly different (P>0.05, Figure 4-4-1).

Compared with the control group, the integrin β2 expression in VTE group increased significantly (P<0.05). Compared with the control group, in different risk factor groups (acute infection, malignancy, autoimmune diseases and trauma/ surgery), the integrin β2 expression was not significantly different (P>0.05, see Figure 4-4-1).

Compared with the control group, the integrin β3 expression in VTE group was significantly elevated (P<0.05). However, the integrin β3 expression levels in different

Table 4-4-1　Baseline data of 1006 subjects

Variables	Group	VTE N=72	INF N=330	CAN N=144	IMD N=103	SUR N=111	CONTROL N=246	TOTAL N=1006
Age	Mean±SD	64.86±15.58	76.15±12.80	67.36±12.67	56.86±14.22	51.07±18.72	68.35±13.62	67.40±16.26
Gender	Male(%)	32(44.44)	196(59.39)	90(62.50)	19(18.63)	69(62.16)	128(52.03)	534(53.08)
	Female(%)	44(55.56)	134(40.61)	54(37.50)	83(81.37)	42(37.84)	118(47.97)	472(46.92)
$\beta1$	Mean±SD	13.42±5.22	11.37±6.39	12.34±5.40	11.48±5.45	10.24±6.33	9.74±4.62	11.15±5.76
	Low (n, %)	1(1.39)	18(5.45)	0(0.00)	2(1.96)	5(4.50)	7(2.85)	33(3.28)
	Normal (n, %)	40(55.56)	214 (64.85)	95(65.97)	68 (66.67)	85(76.58)	206(83.74)	708(70.45)
	High (n, %)	31(43.06)	98(29.70)	49 (34.03)	32(31.37)	21(18.92)	33(13.41)	264(26.27)
$\beta2*$	Median	94.70(76.30,98.71)	91.9(87.50,98.80)	91.40(76.90,98.50)	91.10(75.20,98.60)	91.00(71.90,98.40)	90.50(75.60,97.90)	91.40(75.20,98.60)
	Low (n, %)	1(1.45)	20(6.27)	2(1.40)	3(3.19)	6(5.41)	9(3.67)	41(4.18)
	Normal (n, %)	39(56.52)	197(61.76)	109(76.22)	62 (65.96)	89(80.18)	202(82.45)	698(71.15)
	High (n, %)	29 (42.03)	102(31.97)	32 (22.38)	29(30.85)	16 (14.41)	34 (13.88)	242(24.67)
$\beta3$	Mean±SD	11.05±4.05	9.79±4.07	10.33±3.55	10.21±4.03	8.74±2.43	9.27±3.02	9.76±3.64
	Low (n, %)	1(1.39)	21(6.36)	2(1.39)	4(3.92)	3(2.70)	12(4.88)	43(4.28)
	Normal (n, %)	57(79.17)	272(82.42)	124(86.11)	87(85.29)	107(96.40)	226(91.87)	873 (86.87)
	High (n, %)	14 (19.44)	37(11.21)	18 (12.50)	11(10.78)	1 (0.90)	8(3.25)	89(8.86)

*indicating non normal distribution

[Control value rang] β1:3.14-13.90; β2: 73.40-95.30; β3: 4.39-14.71

risk factor groups (acute infection, malignancy, autoimmune diseases, trauma/ surgery) were not significantly different (P>0.05, see Figure 4-4-1).

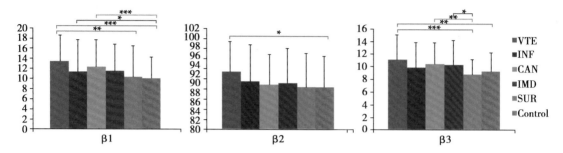

Figure 4-4-1   (1) there is significant difference between VTE(INF, CAN, IMD)and control group for ß1, VTE and SUR group for ß1. (2) there is significant difference between VTE and control group for ß2. (3) there is significant difference between VTE and control group for ß3. VTE and (SUR) group for ß3 *indicating: P<0.05; **indicating: P<0.01; *** indicating: $P<0.001$(American Journal Of Translational Research,2015,7(3):624-631)

The principal findings in this study are firstly that there is an increased expression of integrins β1, β2 and β3 in patients with VTE. Secondly, in most patient groups traditionally considered at risk of VTE (infection, inflammation and malignancy) there was increased expression of β1 but not of β2 or β3. However this increased expression was not found in patients following trauma or surgery, calling into question that such patients are at increased VTE risk in the absence of other factors such as concomitant infection.

Integrins are cell adhesion receptors, which play an important role in the interaction between cells and extracellular matrix (ECM), and in cell-cell interactions [1]. Integrins are heterodimers consisting of noncovalently linked α and β transmembrane glycoprotein subunits. They consist of at least 18 α and 8 β subunits, producing 24 different heterodimers [2]. The α and β subunits separate from each other once the integrin is activated, and then the α subunit binds the ligand. The β1 subunit is expressed mainly on cell surface of lymphocytes, and its ligands consist of laminins, collagens, thrombospondin, vascular cell adhesion molecule 1 and fibronectin [2, 3]. The β2 subunit is distributed on cell surface of neutrophils and monocytes, and ligands for this subunit include fibrinogen, complement component iC3b, intracellular adhesion molecule-1, factor X and so on[4,5]. The β3 subunit is observed on platelets, and this subunit binds fibrinogen, fibronectin, vitronectin von Willebrand factor (vWF) and thrombospondin [6,7].

Integrin β1 is mainly expressed on lymphocytes, and increased integrin β1 expression is related to the inflammation, thrombosis, homing of lymphocytes and metastasis of cancer cells. Integrin β2 is mainly distributed on neutrophils and monocytes, and increased integrin β2 expression is associated with inflammation.

Integrin β3 is mainly expressed on platelets, and elevated integrin β3 expression suggests the platelet activation which is associated with platelet aggregation and thrombosis.

The study results showed that the expression of integrins β1, β2 and β3 increased significantly in VTE group, and integrin β1 elevated markedly in risk factor groups (acute infection, malignancy and autoimmune diseases), but that of integrin β2 or β3 had no significant difference in all risk factor groups. This suggests that there was difference in the protein expression between VTE group and risk factor groups. The elevated expression of integrins β2 and β3 suggests the activation of neutrophils, monocytes and platelets, which is a basic process in the inflammation and thrombosis. Thus, we speculate that the risk factor groups have activated lymphocytes immune cells, and the VTE group may have activated lymphocytes, neutrophils and platelets. The trauma/ surgery group may have no activation of immune cells and platelets and so may not be the "true" risk factor for VTE.

In the present study, the elevated expression of integrins β1, β2 and β3 in VTE group patients was highly consistent with the findings from immunohistochemistry of red thrombus in acute PE patients. In the risk factor groups, those with acute infection, malignancy or autoimmune diseases have increased expression of integrin β1,but the expression of integrins β2 and β3 had no significant difference. This suggests that there is expression difference of core proteins of red thrombus between VTE group and risk factor groups (acute infection, malignancy or autoimmune diseases, trauma/ surgery). In the screening of VTE patients, the increased expression of integrin β1 suggests the elevated risk for venous thrombosis, so prevention against VTE should be done in these patients. The increased expression of integrins β1, β2 and β3 has a value in the clinical diagnosis of VTE. The detection of the expression of integrins β1, β2 and β3 is helpful to diagnose VTE and screen risk people, thus, integrins β1, β2 and β3 may serve as new specific protein markers of VTE and risk people.

The current work is based on the previous studies on genomics [8], proteomics [9], bioinformatics and venous thrombosis core protein screened by immunohistochemstry [10,11]. The present study aimed to verify the core protein in VTE group and risk factor groups. Due to the limitations of sample size in our study, further larger-size or multi-central studies on the normal range of the venous thrombosis core protein are still needed.

(published: Am J Transl Res 2015;7(3):624-631)

References

1. Barczyk M, Carracedo S, Gullberg D. Integrins. Cell Tissue Res 2010;339:269-280.
2. Cavers M, Afzali B, Macey M, McCarthy DA, Irshad S, Brown KA. Differential expression of beta1 and beta2

integrins and L-selectin on CD_4 and CD_8 T lymphocytes in human blood: comparative analysis between isolated cells, whole blood samples and cryopreserved preparations. Clin Exp Immunol. 2002 Jan;127(1):60-5.

3. Fiorilli P, Partridge D, Staniszewska I, Wang JY, Grabacka M, So K, Marcinkiewicz C, Reiss K, Khalili K, Croul SE. Integrins mediate adhesion of medulloblastoma cells to tenascin and activate pathways associated with survival and proliferation. Lab Invest. 2008 Nov;88(11):1143-56.

4. Rezzonico R, Chicheportiche R, Imbert V, Dayer JM. Engagement of CD11b and CD11c beta2 integrin by antibodies or soluble CD23 induces IL-1beta production on primary human monocytes through mitogen-activated protein kinase-dependent pathways. Blood. 2000;95(12):3868-77.

5. Schwarz M, Nordt T, Bode C, Peter K. The GP IIb/IIIa inhibitor abciximab (c7E3) inhibits the binding of various ligands to the leukocyte integrin Mac-1 (CD11b/CD18, alphaMbeta2). Thromb Res. 2002 Aug 15;107(3-4):121-8.

6. Fang J, Nurden P, North P, Nurden AT, Du LM, Valentin N, Wilcox DA. C560Rβ3 caused platelet integrin αII b β3 to bind fibrinogen continuously, but resulted in a severe bleeding syndrome and increased murine mortality. J Thromb Haemost. 2013 Jun;11(6):1163-71. doi: 10.1111/jth.12209.

7. Coburn J, Magoun L, Bodary SC, Leong JM. Integrins alpha(v)beta3 and alpha5beta1 mediate attachment of lyme disease spirochetes to human cells. Infect Immun. 1998 May;66(5):1946-52.

8. Xie Y, Duan Q, Wang L, Gong Z, Wang Q, Song H, Wang H. Genomic characteristics of adhesion molecules in patients with symptomatic pulmonary embolism. Mol Med Rep 2012;6:585-590.

9. Wang L, Gong Z, Jiang J, Xu W, Duan Q, Liu J,Qin C. Confusion of wide thrombolytic time window for acute pulmonary embolism: mass spectrographic analysis for thrombus proteins. Am J Respir Crit Care Med. 2011;184:145-146.

10. Wang LM, Duan QL, Yang F, Yi XH, Zeng Y, Tian HY, Lv W, Jin Y. Activation of circulated immune cells and inflammatory immune adherence are involved in the whole process of acute venous thrombosis Int J Clin Exp Me 2014;7(3):566-572

11. LeMin Wang, Qiang-Lin Duan1, Xiang-Hua Yi, Yu Zeng, Zhu Gong1, Fan Yang.Venous thromboembolism is a product in proliferation of cancer cells Int J Clin Exp Med 2014;7(5):1319-1323

Chapter 5

Venous thrombus and pathogenic microorganism

1. Severe Acute Respiratory Syndrome and VTE in multiple organs

Severe Acute Respiratory Syndrome (SARS) is now known to be caused by a novel coronavirus, the SARS-associated coronavirus (SARS-CoV) [1], and is characterized by severe systemic symptoms in multi-organs such as lung, immune system, and small vessels, etc., finally leading to respiratory failure. Initial autopsies reported the predominant pathological findings to be diffuse lung damages, injured immune organs, inflammatory responses in systemic small vessels and general toxic reactions [2]. Changes in coagulation and the development of thrombi have been reported in patients with SARS but the extent of the effects of the SARS-associated coronavirus on the systemic circulation has yet to be established. Limited data are available on the extent of the damage to the systemic vasculature and circulation in patients with SARS. In the present study, an autopsy was performed on a 57-year-old man diagnosed with SARS and specimens from multiple organs were analyzed to assess pathological changes in the vasculature. Specimens from multiple organs, including the lungs, heart, liver, kidneys, adrenal glands, spleen, esophagus, stomach, intestine, appendices vermicularis, pancreas, brain, cerebellum, brainstem, hilus of lung, mesenteric lymph node and muscle tissues were analyzed by light microscopy. Examination of all of the specimens revealed systemic circulatory disturbance and polyangiitis. proliferation, swelling, and apoptosis of endothelial cells, and edema, inflammatory cell infiltration, and fibrinoid necrosis were observed in the walls of small blood vessels in specimens from the lungs, heart, liver, kidneys, adrenal glands, brain, gastrointestinal tract, and muscle tissues. In addition, thrombi were evident in the veins and microcirculation of the soft tissues surrounding the lungs, spleen, pancreas, kidneys, adrenal glands, and mesenteric lymph nodes (Figure 5-1-1 A-F).

This autopsy case report demonstrated that in addition to the well established diffuse alveolar damage and damage to the immune system, SARS is associated with systemic circulatory disturbance and polyangiitis, in particular thrombosis, in the veins and microcirculation in multiple organs and tissues. To our knowledge, this is the first

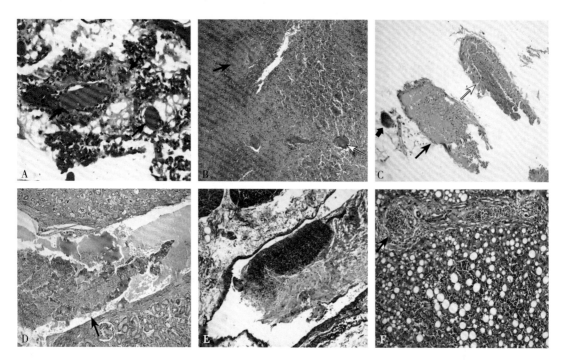

Figure 5-1-1(A-F)   The multiple organs autopsy of a SARS patient. (A). Lung: thrombi in the lumen of the small vessels (arrow) and significant pulmonary edema and hemorrhage. HE×200; (B)Spleen: thickening and hyaline degeneration of the splenic central artery (solid arrow); and the hyaline thrombi in small vessels (open arrow). HE×40; (C)Lymphatic system: thrombosis within small vessels in the soft tissue surrounding the mesenteric lymph nodes: hyaline thrombus (thick arrow), mixed thrombus (thin arrow) and red thrombus (open arrow). HE×100; (D) Renal interstitium: mixed thrombi (arrow) composed of fibrin, platelets and red blood cells. HE×40; (E)Pancreatic lobular interstitium: aggregation of white blood cells and fibrin clot, incomplete occlusion in the vascular cavity (arrow) and perivascular interstitial edema. HE×40; (F)Liver: Vascular dilatation and congestion in the peri-portal region are shown (arrow). HE×100. (American Journal Of Respiratory And Critical Care Medicine,2010,182: 436-437)

study to show the extent of the damage to the vasculature and circulation that can occur in patients with SARS.

DVT and/or PE have been reported in patients with SARS previously [3-4]. However, the pathogenesis of DVT in patients with SARS remains unknown. Emerging evidence suggests that viral infection may have a role in the onset of venous thromboembolism [5-6]. The present study adds to this evidence by demonstrating widespread thrombosis associated with SARS.

(published: Am J Respir Crit Care Med. Aug 1 2010;182(3):436-437).

2. Virus-like structure in a patient with pulmonary hypertension and VTE

HIV infection has been widely recognized as one of the causes for the pathogenesis of pulmonary arterial hypertension [1,2]. In a previous study of HIV-related pulmonary hypertension (HRPH), authors pointed out that the pathogenesis of HIV-PAH is believed to be associated with viral proteins such as Nef, Tat and gp120 [3]. HIV-1 Nef protein perhaps in conjunction with persistent immune dysregulation contributes to the development of pulmonary vasculatures remodeling by inducing secretion of inflammatory cytokines [4]. However, whether other types of virus, especially those which cannot be routinely identified in clinical practice, can also play an important role in the pathogenesis of PAH or has not been investigated so far. At the same time, there has been little direct evidence of the pathogens' action during the pathogenic process of PAH. Therefore, we here report a case of previously healthy 11-year-old girl diagnosed as PAH 3 months after upper respiratory tract infection caused by undetermined virus. Thirteen months after diagnosis of PAH, the girl died of right heart failure. Blood test revealed the increase of D-Dimer which indicated the possibility of embolism in this patient. Immunophenotyping showed that function of T cell immunity was compromised with the decreased cell count of CD_3 (50.7% ↓, normal value 60-85%) and CD_8 (17.8% ↓ , 18.5-42.1%) but with normal cell count of CD_4 (29.0%, 24.5-48.8%). In addition, we also found the same phenomenon in other 6 of 8 (75%) patients with chronic thromboembolic pulmonary hypertension when performing T cell immunity test in 30 PE patients with or without PAH. Meanwhile, several enveloped mulberry-like structures were detected in the cytoplasm of T lymphocytes, accompanied by budding and proliferation under electron microscopy observation. The size of these structures is similar to virus. The dynamic process of adhering to and departing from T lymphocytes for these structures was in line with the process of virus pullulation and release to and from T cells (Figure 5-2-1). Thus, we supposed that the compromised T cell mediated immunity function is associated with the infection of these virus-like structures with the exclusion of other causes clinically in this patient.

We previously showed that T cell immunity function associated genes were down-regulated in patients with pulmonary embolism by means of gene profiling analyses [5]. Therefore, we hypothesize that not only the HIV infection but also other types of viral infections might lead to pulmonary hypertension through deteriorating host T cell immunity function and ensuing events. This special case offers clinical clue for the studies on the etiology of pulmonary hypertension and need to be further verified.

(published: Am J Respir Crit Care Med. 2010; 182(3): 434-435).

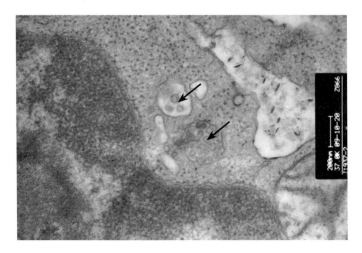

Figure 5-2-1A   Round structures with intact capsules and different densities of granules in the cytoplasm of T cells (↑, *37,000) (American Journal Of Respiratory And Critical Care Medicine,2010,182: 434-435)

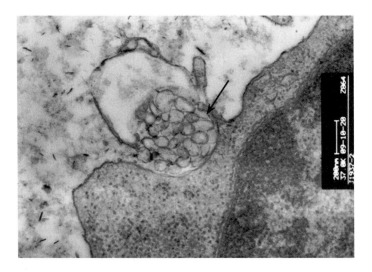

Figure 5-2-1B   Mulberry-like pathogenic microorganisms penetrated through the T-cell membrane and pullulated (↑ *37,000) (American Journal Of Respiratory And Critical Care Medicine,2010,182: 434-435)

Reference

1. Aarons, E.J. and F.J. Nye, Primary pulmonary hypertension and HIV infection. AIDS, 1991. 5(10): p. 1276-7.

2. Sitbon, O., et al., Prevalence of HIV-related pulmonary arterial hypertension in the current antiretroviral therapy era. Am J Respir Crit Care Med, 2008. 177(1): p. 108-13.

3. Marecki, J.C., et al., HIV-1 Nef is associated with complex pulmonary vascular lesions in SHIV-nef-infected

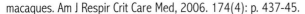

macaques. Am J Respir Crit Care Med, 2006. 174(4): p. 437-45.

4. Hassoun, P.M., et al., Inflammation, growth factors, and pulmonary vascular remodeling. J Am Coll Cardiol, 2009. 54(1 Suppl): p. S10-9.

5. Gong Zhu, Liang Ai-bin, Wang le-min, et al. The expression and significance of imuunity associated genes mRNA in patients with pulmonary embolism[J].Chin J Intern Med,2009,48(8),666-669.

3. Bacteremia and the occurrence of VTE in multiple organs

Venous thromboembolism (VTE) including acute pulmonary embolism (APE), chronic thromboembolic pulmonary hypertension (CTEPH) and deep venous thrombosis (DVT) is a global disease. The high morbidity, high misdiagnosis rate and high mortality render PE as a worldwide health problem. Smeeth et al reported that acute infection was closely related to the occurrence of VTE, especially within 2 weeks after infection [1]. Pathogenic microorganisms such as viruses, bacteria and parasites can invade the body and cause infective inflammation; however, the immune defensive mechanism of human body against various microorganisms is different. Bacterial toxins can activate neutrophils, monocytes, macrophages, lymphocytes and endothelial cells in a certain order, and these cells will produce a variety of factors including pro-inflammatory cytokines, and express various adhesion molecules [2].

A 52-year-old male developed PE and DVT in the lower extremity one week after diagnosis of acute enteritis. The symptoms alleviated after treatment, but VTE relapsed repeatedly. This patient was again admitted to hospital due to DVT in the lower extremity 6 months later. Peripheral blood was collected. Electron microscopy showed that neutrophils were apoptotic rod-shaped, and bacteria-like microorganisms were identified in the vacuolus cavity of neutrophils (Figure 5-3-1 A, B, C, D). The presence of rod-shaped bacteria-like microorganisms in neutrophils indicates immune dysfunction or immune suppression of neutrophils in VTE patients with bacteremia.

To overcome immune imbalance, the body will mobilize and activate other immune cells. Under the stimulation of infective agents, white blood cells, platelets and endothelial cells will be activated and the expression of integrins on the surface of membrane will be increased. The integrins with conformational changes can bind the ligand fibrinogen to generate the thrombus protein network, leading to the occurrence of VTE. Viral infection has been reported to be closely related to the occurrence of VTE [3,4]. The relationship between bacterial infection and VTE that we reported previously suggests that various pathogen infections may be the etiological factors in the occurrence of VTE.

In the surface of some bacteria, viruses and parasites, there exists similar structure

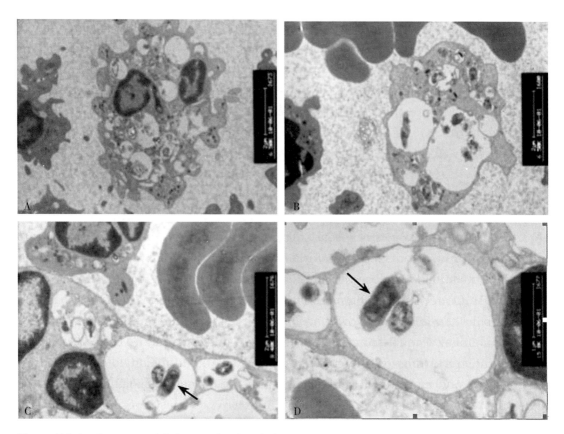

Figure 5-3-1   the neutrophil damage and pod-shaped bacteria-like microorganisms under electron microscope. A: Apoptotic neutrophils; B: The nucleus of neutrophils disappeared; C: pod-shaped bacteria-like microorganisms were identified in the cytoplasmic cavity of phagocytes(arrow); D: pod-shaped bacteria-like microorganisms at a higher magnification (arrow). (American Journal Of Respiratory And Critical Care Medicine,2012,186: 696)

of the adhesion molecule ligand, which can bind integrin on the surface of membrane protein to mediate cell adhesion response when cells are infected [5], and the binding may also be directly involved in venous thrombosis.

(published: Am J Respir Crit Care Med. 2012; 186(7): 696).

References

1. Smeeth L, Cook C, Thomas S, Hall AJ, Hubbard R, Vallance P. Risk of deep vein thrombosis and pulmonary embolism after acute infection in a community setting. Lancet. 2006, 367(9516): 1075-1079.

2. König B, Köller M, Prevost G, Piemont Y, Alouf JE, Schreiner A, König W. Activation of human effector cells by different bacterial toxins (leukocidin, alveolysin, and erythrogenic toxin A): generation of interleukin-8. Infect Immun.1994;62(11):4831-7.

3. Xiang-Hua Y, Le-Min W, Ai-Bin L, Zhu G, Riquan L, Xu-You Z, Wei-Wei R, Ye-Nan W. Severe acute respiratory syndrome and venous thromboembolism in multiple organs. Am J Respir Crit Care Med. Aug 1 2010;182(3):436-437.

4. Wang L, Gong Z, Liang A, Xie Y, Liu SL, Yu Z, Wang L, Wang Y. Compromised T-cell immunity and virus-like structure in a patient with pulmonary hypertension. Am J Respir Crit Care Med. 2010;182(3):434-435.

5. Pribila JT, Quale AC, Mueller KL, Shimizu Y. Integrins and T cell-mediated immunity. Annu Rev Immunol. 2004;22:157-80.

Chapter 6

Function and regulation of the immune system

1. Immune function

The immune system is composed of immune tissues, immune organs, immune cells and immune active molecules, which together implement the immune defense and keep the body fit through collaborating harmoniously to recognize and eliminate the external invasive pathogens and internal senile cells and malignant cells. Simply speaking, it is the function of the immune system that removes all the foreign agents inside human body, including external pathogenic microorganism, implants, invasive foreign bodies and toxins from wounds; and internally generated senile cells and malignant cells. Through a long-term evolutionary process, the immune system with both inside and outside functions has developed perfect tissue structures and exceptional functions. Immune organs, which mainly consist of lymphatic tissues, distribute widely all over the body, including central immune organs and peripheral immune organs. Among them, the thymus and bone marrow both belong to the central organs in immune system.

The immune system can be divided into innate immune system and adaptive immune system. The innate immunity, also called congenital immunity, is the oldest existing functionality in the biological evolution, which eliminates the encountered foreign bodies immediately through its components, including macrophages, granulocytes, natural killer cells and complement system. However, the adaptive immunity is acquired after birth with a characteristic of having memories, which can specifically attack the same invasive foreign agents. That is why the adaptive immunity is also named specific immunity, which functions mainly through T and B lymphocytes.

As the three major systems in human body, immune system, nervous system and endocrine system play important roles in regulating human physical activities and self-balance. Innate and adaptive immunities are mediated by vegetative nerves and endocrines, among which vegetative nerves regulate the phagocytes or lymphocytes into their perfect status. Hormones can regulate the immune function levels between tissues. Under strong stress, the functioning immune system switches. The increased adrenocortical hormones inhibit the T and B lymphocytes for a short time and activate the immune system of T lymphocytes differentiated outside thymus. Cytokines regulate the cooperation between immune cells and interactions between lymphocytes or between phagocytes and lymphocytes to promote cell growth and inhibit cell functions. The immune balance is a complicated process. Different immune functioning status determines different body status. Immune function inhibition or immune system collapse indicates that immune cells in the innate and adaptive system has a state of no function or significant dysfunction. Short-term inhibition of immune cell functions presents periodic collapse of immune cell function, while durative collapse will lead to irreversible diseases.

2. Factors affecting immune cell functions

(1) Age increase
The immune system does not completely establish in neonates but becomes mature and immune function improves with age. The immune function peaks at age of 20-30 years and thereafter reduces over age.

(2) Stress
Highly evolved, complicated immune system is regulated by the autonomic nervous system. Autonomic nervous system is a regulatory center of the immune system network, and the center of autonomic nervous system is the brain. Autonomic nerves are derived from the brain and extend all over the body including the sites around the blood vessels. Besides the regulation by the autonomic nervous system, the immune system also cooperates with endocrine system to regulate the immune function. Nervous system, endocrine system and immune system are three important systems in humans and play crucial roles in the physiological activities and homeostasis. Innate immunity and adaptive immunity are modulated by the autonomic nervous system and endocrine system, and the autonomic nervous system may also regulate the systemic phagocytes or lymphocytes and determinate the preponderant function of different types of cells. Steroids regulate the immune function among tissues. Under intense stress, the immune functions of T and B cells are transiently inhibited, and the differentiation of extrathymic T cells is initiated. Cytokines may regulate the cooperation of immune cells as well as the interaction between phagocytes and lymphocytes.

(3) Food balance
The production of immune cells and the synthesis of immunoreactive substances have involvement of raw materials including nutrients and trace elements. There is also a relationship between trace elements and immune functions. The basic elements composing lives are carbon, hydrogen, oxygen and nitrogen (account for 90%), while

the rest are sulfur, phosphorus, potassium, sodium, calcium, chloride, magnesium, iron and so on (accounting for more than 9%). The contents of the elements such as zinc, selenium, copper, chromium, iodine, iron as well as manganese are extremely low, which are called trace elements. Nevertheless, trace elements, which are related to physical strength, intelligence, diseases and lifetime, play important roles in maintaining normal metabolism. They are involved in synthesis of various kinds of enzymes, nucleic acids and proteins, and elevating and regulating immune functions including innate immunity, cellular immunity and humoral immunity. Trace elements can only be supplied from outside and the insufficiency of trace elements may influence and compromise the immune function.

(4) Environmental factors

Human and nature are an organic unity. Ecological balance is the guarantee of healthy society. Environmental factors including air, water, sunshine, soil, vegetation, house, social humanity and so on, directly impact immune cell function of the body. In addition, the number of immune cells changes between day and night and over seasons, body temperature and age.

Vegetative nerve consists of sympathetic nerves that are dominant in daytime and parasympathetic nerves that are dominant at night. Thus, with the changes of day and night, the defensive methods of white blood cells change also. The percentage of granulocytes increases in the daytime, going up from 4:00 a.m., peaking at noon and then going down, while that of lymphocytes increases at night, hitting the rock bottom at noon, going up to the peak at 4:00 a.m. and going down again. The rule of white blood cell changes through day and night is the result of biological evolution.

Immune cells can be influenced by changes of atmospheric pressure and the season. As the atmospheric pressure, air temperature, humidity and season change, the functions of vegetative nerves and immune system undergo a large correction. The sympathetic nerves preponderate under the circumstance of low air temperature and humidity, while the parasympathetic nerves preponderate under the circumstance of high air temperature and humidity. Due to the high oxygen content, the sympathetic nerves preponderate under high atmospheric pressure; on the contrary, the parasympathetic nerves preponderate under low atmospheric pressure. The atmospheric pressure varies a lot with seasons, thus vegetative nerves differ a lot with seasons also. In winter, low air temperature and high atmospheric pressure make the sympathetic nerves dominant, whereas in summer, the parasympathetic nerves become dominant. Without doubt, the proportion of white blood cells changes as regulation of the vegetative nerves.

Body temperature also has impacts on immune cells. The body temperature keeps vibrating in the daytime and is controlled by the vegetative nerves. The average core temperature is 37.2°C in normal people, at which the enzymes are most active inside human body. The lymphocytes are apt to be activated at high body temperature, while malignant cell are apt to differentiate and proliferate at low body temperature. What's more, the functions of mitochondria are inhibited when the body temperature is low.

References

Immunology Lecture by professor TORU ABO 2010 Sanwa co.Ltd

General theory of genomics in patients with symptomatic pulmonary thromboembolism (PE)

The charactritics of human genomics are wholeness, comprehensiveness and direction. There are differences in the protein expression guided by gene expression, so the results should be verified by proteomics and cytology. Intro-group comparison of genomic expression profile and functional analysis of significantly different profiles provide the wholeness and direction of understanding diseases, which is not processed by other meansures.

1. Pandect—Network analysis of human genome differences

Human genomics has the advantages of wholeness, comprehensiveness and directionality. Although the gene guided synthesis of proteins varies among proteins, and proteinology and cytology are usually required for validation, the comparisons of genomics expression patterns between groups and functional analysis of differentially expressed proteins may provide the wholeness and directionality for the understanding of pathogenesis of disease. This is a global detection that other methods do no possess. This study aimed to display the global gene expression profiles in pulmonary thromboembolism (PE) patients.

Methods: PE patients and controls matched in age and gender were recruited into present study, and malignancies and autoimmune diseases were excluded. PE was diagnosed according to the clinical manifestations and imaging examinations. Acute arterial or venous thrombosis was excluded in the control group. Whole-genome expression analysis and Gene Ontology analysis were employed, and small sample t-test after repeated correction, functional analysis of differentially expressed genes and path-net analysis of differentially expressed genes were used for statistical analysis.

Results: 1) GO analysis showed that the genes with significant down-regulation were related to the immune receptor complex and immune function of T cells in PE patients; 2) functional analysis of differentially expressed genes and t-test showed that the mRNA expressions of genes related to phagocytes and adhesion molecules were significantly up-regulated in PE patients; 3) path-net analysis indicated that the pathogenesis of PE was associated with microorganism infection and compromised immunity; 4) The mRNA expressions of genes related to vascular endothelial cells and coagulation remained unchanged in PE patients, and the mRNA expressions of several genes associated with anti-coagulation system, fibrinolytic system and platelet function changed signifiantly.

The expression of genes related to the immune function of T cells is significantly down-regulated and the mRNA expression of adhesion molecules is markedly up-regulated in symptomatic VTE patients. These findings imply that VTE is an inflammatory process due to compromised cellular immunity.

(Published: Mol Med Rep 2015; 11: 2527-2533).

2. Systematics of genomics

Phagocytic cells, NK cells, the complement system, T cells and B cells are important participants of innate and adaptive immunity. Each of them possesses the ability to defend against pathogens and they act together to form immune defense. Overall, genomics studies indicate that the expressions of phagocytic cells related genes are significantly up-regulated, but those of NK cells related genes are markedly down-regulated, the expressions of compliments relate genes are disordered, there is an evident imbalance in the expressions of cytokines related genes, the expressions of T cells related genes are significantly down-regulated, the expressions of B cells related genes are disorganized in PE patients. In patients with symptomatic PE, there is acute inflammatory response and the systemic immune cell balance is disrupted.

Expression characteristics of neutrophil and mononuclear-phagocyte related genes in patients with PE

Human genomics characteristics of phagocytes between clinically symptomatic pulmonary thromboembolism (PE) and controls were systematically compared to explore the innate immunologic pathogenesis of PE.

Methods: Twenty patients with symptomatic PE and 20 sex- and age-matched subjects without PE as controls were enrolled in our study. mRNA expressions of genes related to phagocytes were analyzed by means of microarray.

Results: In comparison with controls, mRNA expressions of phagocytes pattern recognition receptors and opsonic receptors were totally up-regulated, among which TLR4, CD14, MYD88, SCARB2, SCARF2, FCGR2A and CR1 were markedly up-regulated (P <0.01).

In symptomatic PE patients, phagocytes are excessively activated, which indicates that abnormal immunity and inflammatory response induced by activated phagocytes may be one of the mechanisms of the occurrence of symptomatic PE.

(published:Mol Med Rep 2015; 11: 2527-2533)

Expression characteristics of natural killer cell related genes in patients with PE

To investigate the role of natural killer cells in the pathogenesis of PE.

Methods: Twenty patients with PE were enrolled in our study and the other 20 patients without PE were allocated as control. Total RNA was abstracted from isolated mononuclear cells, which include natural killer cells in peripheral blood samples of 20 patients and controls. Significantly differential mRNA expressions of natural killer cell receptor gene were analyzed by means of mRNA expression microarray.

Results: Twenty-one mRNA fragments associated with receptors of NK cells were screened. In comparison with control, the mRNA expressions of C-type lectin superfamily receptors, KIR and NCR in PTE group were down expressed compared to control. mRNA expression of NCR1 and C-type lectin superfamily receptors were remarkably down-regulated in 78% gene investigated (P<0.05); the mRNA expression of CD11a and CD_{16} gene was significantly up-regulated (P<0.05).

NK cells were inhibited in the process of PTE. Up-regulated mRNA expression of CD11a and CD_{16} indicated that the adhering activity of NK cell and antibody-dependent cell- mediated cytotoxicity was enhanced. Generally, NK cell is involved in the process of PE formation.

(published:Int J Clin Exp Pathol 2015;8(7):8244-8251)

Expression characteristics of complement system related genes mRNA in patients with PE

Twenty cases of PE patients and twenty sex and age matched controls were recruited into the study. Human cDNA microarray analysis was used to detect the gene expression difference of the complement system between the two groups.

Results: 1).Expression of twenty-one genes encoding complement components was detected. In PE patients,expression of the genes encoding C1qα, C1qβ, C4b, C5 and Factor P was significantly greater (P<0.05) than controls, while C6, C7, C9, mannose-binding lectin (MBL) and mannan-binding lectin serine peptidase 1 (MASP1) mRNAs were lower (P<0.05) than controls. 2)Expression of seven genes encoding complement receptors was examined. In PE patients, CR1, integrin αM, integrin αX and C5aR mRNAs were significantly up-regulated (P<0.01) compared with controls. 3) Seven genes encoding complement regulators were examined. The mRNA expression of CD59 and CD55 was significantly up-regulated (P<0.05), whereas Factor I mRNA was significantly down-regulated (P<0.05) in PE patients than controls.

In PE patients, the mRNA expressions of complement components, receptors and regulators were unbalanced, suggesting dysfunction and/or deficiency of the complement system, which leads to decreased function of MAC-induced cell lysis in PE patients finally.

(published:Thromb Res 2013;132:e54-7).

Expression characteristics of Cytokine related genes mRNA in patients with PE

Twenty patients with PE and twenty control patients matched for gender and age with the PE group were recruited into the study. Human cDNA microarray analysis was used to detect differences in the expression of cytokine-associated genes between the two groups.

Results: In PE patients, the expression levels of the genes encoding IFNα5, IFNα6, IFNα8, IFNα14, IFNκ, IFNω1, IFNε1 and IFNγ were significantly lower compared with controls (P<0.05). The expression levels of the genes encoding IL1α, IL2, IL3, IL9, IL13, IL17β, IL19, IL22, IL23α, IL24, IL25 and IL31 were significantly lower (P<0.05), while IL10 and IL28A mRNA expression levels were higher in PE patients compared with controls (P<0.05). In PE patients, Cxcl1, Cxcl2, Cxcl6, Cxcl13 and Cxcl14 mRNAs were significantly upregulated (P<0.05), however, Cxcl10 mRNA was significantly downregulated (P<0.01). In PE patients, the mRNA expression levels of TNF superfamily members 1, 9 and 13, and TNF receptor superfamily members 1A, 1B, 9, 10B, 10C, 10D and 19L, were significantly upregulated (P<0.05), whereas TNF receptor superfamily members 11B, 19 and 25 were significantly downregulated compared with controls (P<0.05). The mRNA expression levels of granulocyte-macrophage colony-stimulating factor, granulocyte colony-stimulating factor, erythropoietin, thrombopoietin and mast cell growth factor were significantly lower in PE patients compared with controls (P<0.05). In PE patients, the mRNA expression levels of a variety of cytokines were imbalanced and cellular immune function was downregulated compared with controls.

(published:Mol Med Rep 2013;7:124)

Expression characteristics of adhesion molecules related genes in patients with PE

Whole human gene chip was applied to detect the expression of cell adhesion molecule-related mRNAs in symptomatic PE and in the control group, and statistical analysis was performed.

Results: In patients with PE, the expression of the majority of integrin mRNAs located on leukocytes and platelets was significantly upregulated. The expression of mRNAs related to L-selectin and P-selectin glycoprotein ligand was significantly upregulated, while the expression of mRNA related to E-selectin was significantly downregulated. The expression of mRNAs related to classic cadherins and protocadherins was downregulated, and the expression of mRNAs related to vascular endothelial cadherin was significantly downregulated; the expression of mRNAs related to the immunoglobulin superfamily had no obvious difference between the two groups.

In symptomatic PE patients, the adhesion of leukocytes and platelets was enhanced; the activation of endothelial cells was obviously weakened; the adherens junctions among endothelial cells were weakened, with the endothelium becoming more permeable.

(published:Mol Med Rep 2012;6:585-90).

The Differential Expression of Leucocyte β2 Integrins Signal Transduction Associated Genes in Patients with PE

Whole human genome oligo microarrays were employed to systematically investigate the differential expression characteristics of associated mRNAs, which were found in the signal transduction pathway of β2 integrins in peripheral blood mononuclear cells (PBMCs) between patients with symptomatic pulmonary thromboembolism (PE) and controls. A total of 20 cases of PE patients and twenty gender-and age-matched controls were recruited for the study. Human cDNA microarray analysis was used to detect the differences in mRNA expression between the two groups and a random variance model corrected t-test was used to analyze the statistical data. A total of 80 associated mRNAs were detected.

Results: The mRNA expression of chemokines, ligands, inside-out and outside-in signaling pathway-associated proteins were upregulated significantly in the PE group, compared with the controls. In five subunit-associated mRNAs, the mRNA expression of ITGAL, ITGAM, ITGAX and ITGB2, which encode the subunits of αL, αM, αX and β2, were upregulated in the PE group and the differences, with the exception of ITGB2, were statistically significant ($P<0.05$). The mRNA expression of ITGAD was downregulated; however, there was no significant difference ($P>0.05$). The expression of Fgr mRNA was significantly downregulated ($P<0.01$).

In PE patients, bilateral signal transduction pathways of β2 integrins in neutrophils and monocytes were activated, enhancing innate immunity.

(published:Mol Med Rep 2014;9:285-92).

Analysis on the Pathogenesis of Symptomatic PE with Human Genomics

The characteristics of human genomics and cellular immune function between clinically symptomatic venous thromboembolism (VTE) and controls were systematically compared to explore the immunologic pathogenesis of VTE.

Results: Microarray assay showed that the mRNA expressions of genes related to non-specific cellarer immune and cytokines were significantly down-regulated. Abnormal expressions of CD_3, CD_4, CD_8, NK marker $CD_{16}CD_{56}$, CD_{19} and aberrant CD_4/CD_8 ratio were detected in 54 out of 56 patients. In PE patients, microarray assay revealed the imbalance in the expressions of genes related to the immune system. The expressions of genes related to non-specific immune cells and cytokines were markedly up-regulated and those associated with cellular immune were dramatically down-regulated. In VTE patients, cytological examination indicated that the functions of NK cells were significantly compromised and the antigen recognition and killing function of T cells were markedly decreased.

The consistence between genomic and cytological examination suggests that the symptomatic VTE is closely associated with the infection and immune dysfunction.

(published: Int J Med Sci 2012;9:380-6).

Expression of interleukins and Th1/Th2 imbalance in patients with PE

A total of 20 PE patients and 20 gender- and age-matched controls were included in the study. Human cDNA microarray analysis was used to detect the differences in cytokine gene expression between the two groups and a random variance model corrected t-test was used to analyze the statistical data.

Results: In comparison with the controls, 12 genes were found to be downregulated, specifically IL1A, IL9, IL17B, IL19, IL23A, IL25 (P<0.05), IL2, IL3, IL13, IL22, IL24 and IL31 (P<0.01), and 2 genes were found to be upregulated, specifically IL10 and IL28A, in the PE patients. The expression levels of IFN-γ and IL2 mRNA in the PE patients were significantly lower than those in the control group (P<0.01), while the IL20 mRNA expression levels were significantly upregulated (P<0.01).

There are significant differences in interleukin gene expression between the PE patients and the control group. A shift of the Th1/Th2 balance comprising enhanced Th2 activity and reduced Th1 activity in the PE patients is also demonstrated.

(published:Mol Med Rep 2013;7:332-6.)

Expression characteristics of B cell related genes mRNA in patients with PE

Human complementary DNA microarray analysis was used in order to detect the differential expression of B cell associated genes between the PE and control groups. Messenger (m) RNA expression was detected for 82 genes involved in B cell activation.

Results: PE patients exhibited significantly increased expression levels of the B cell receptor genes LYN, CD22, SYK, BTK, PTPRC and NFAM1, whereas expression levels of FYN, FCRL4 and LAX1 were significantly decreased compared to those of the control group. Expression levels of T cell dependent B cell activation genes, including EMR2, TNFSF9, CD86, ICOSLG, CD37 and CD97, were significantly upregulated in PE patients, whereas SPN mRNA expression was significantly downregulated compared with those of the control group. LILRA1 and TLR9 T cell independent B cell activation mRNAs were significantly upregulated in PE patients compared with those of the control group. In addition, the expression levels of B cell activation regulator genes, including CR1, LILRB4 and VAV1, were significantly increased, whereas SLAMF7 expression levels were significantly decreased in PE patients compared with those of the control group. Furthermore, the expression levels of B cell activation associated cytokine genes demonstrated a significant upregulation of LTA and IL10 and downregulation of L1A, IFNA5, IFNA6, IFNA8, IFNA14, IL2, IL13 and IFNG . The differential gene expression at different stages of B cell activation between controls and PE patients indicated that B cell function was reduced or disorganized in patients with PE.

(published: Mol Med Rep 11: 2299-2305, 2015)

Differential expression of 5-HT-related genes in patients with PE

A total of 20 PE patients and 20 healthy subjects matched in gender and age were recruited. The human genome microarrays were performed to detect the mRNA expression profile of 5-HT synthetase, transporter, receptor, and factors in 5-HT signal pathway of the two groups. The random variance model corrected t-test was used for analysis.

Results: Our results showed (1) tryptophan hydroxylase (TPH1)-related gene expression was markedly down-regulated in PE patients ($P<0.01$); (2) monoamine oxidases (MAO)-related gene (MAOB) expression was significantly up-regulated in PE patients ($P<0.01$); (3) the expression of 17 genes of 7 5-HT receptors showed a down-regulated tendency in PE patients, and significant difference was observed in the expression of HTR1E, HTR3B, HTR4 and HTR5A between them ($P<0.05$); (4) the expression of DalDAG-GEF I, Tubby, PKA and EPAC in5-HT signal pathways was dramatically up-regulated in PE patients ($P<0.05$), whereas the expression of SPA1, RIAM, RAPL, Talin, PKC, PLC and Pyk2 was remarkably up-regulated in PE patients($P<0.05$); (5) the expression of integrin genes ITGA2B, ITGB1 and ITGB3 was significantly up-regulated in PE patients ($P<0.05$).

In PE patients, the expression of TPH1 and HTR4 was down-regulated as a negative feedback; the MAOB expression was up-regulated. Consistent with the expression of 5-HTR1E and 5-HTR4 and the abnormally activated Tubby, the expression of integrins in platelets was activated.

(published: Int J Clin Exp Med 2015;8(1):512-518)

Chapter 8

Characterization of immune cell perforin mutations in a family with VTE

The American College of Chest Physicians (ACCP) has published 9th guidelines for the prevention, diagnosis, and treatment of venous thromboembolism (VTE) from 1995 to 2012 [1]. Risk factors of VTE include infection, malignancies, increasing age, surgery, trauma and family history of VTE, etc. It has been proposed that family history might increase the risk of VTE. A 22-year period study from 1987 to 2009 demonstrated that family history was an important risk factor for VTE, supporting a strong genetic component to VTE [2]. It has been reported that inherited risk factors for VTE are rare and mainly consist of loss-of-function mutations in genes encoding anticoagulant proteins and gain-of-function mutations in genes encoding procoagulant proteins [3].

We have reported that the occurrence of symptomatic VTE was associated with decreased and/or disordered immune function [4]. Transmission electron microscopy showed rod-like bacteria in the phagocytes of a patient with recurrent PE/DVT and virus-like microorganisms in the CD_3 and CD_8T cells of a patient with VTE/PAH, respectively [5,6]. We have reported that a common immunological feature of these patients is that they had decreased number of CD_3 T cells and CD_8T cells, and increased CD_4/CD_8 ratios [7,8]. We have also reported that DVT was found in multiple organs including the lungs, spleen, pancreas, kidneys, and adrenal glands from a patient who died of severe acute respiratory syndrome [9], indicating that virus and bacterial infections were associated with the occurrence of VTE. Infection is a risk factor of VTE, and pathogens invading the body are just an external cause of VTE. However, immune function may be the internal cause of VTE.

We have analyzed the roles of immune cells in the formation of thrombosis in the lung vessels of mice after influenza A/H1N1 infection. To confirm previous clinical findings, an A/H1N1 influenza infection model was established to compare the pulmonary thrombosis in 6 groups of infected mice with different immune statuses (C57BL/6, BALB/c: without deficiency of immune cells; Scid: T, B cells combined deficiency; NOD/LtJ: NK cell deficiency; BALB/c-nu: T cell deficiency; NOD-Scid: T,

B, NK cells combined deficiency). The results showed that the virus could result in thrombosis in pulmonary small arterials, small veins and capillary vessels. In the 4 groups of mice with deficiency of T cells, B cells, NK cells or combined cell deficiency, the incidence rate of thrombosis was significantly greater than that of mice without cellular immune deficiency. Several animal experiments have demonstrated that different types of immune deficiencies can lead to the occurrence of VTE, especially combined immune deficiencies.

Although it has been demonstrated by clinical and animal experiments that pathogenic microorganisms can trigger the occurrence of VTE at the state of immune dysfunction, the sites of immune abnormalities are unclear. In the present study, we carried out exome sequencing in a Chinese Han family with VTE, and it is reported as follows.

Clinical data of this Chinese family

A Han Chinese family (12 members) with VTE was used in this study (Figure 8-1-1A). In the first generation, 2 members (1 with a history of DVT) died; in the second generation, 1 member with a history of DVT died and 3 members were affected; in the third and fourth generation, all 5 members were healthy.

The proband (II:9), a 50-year-old man, presented with right leg swelling at the age of 41. Computed tomography (CT) scan revealed deep vein thrombosis in the right leg. After 1 month of treatment with warfarin, the symptoms disappeared. In 2009, he presented with shortness of breath, cough, and bilateral lower extremity edema but slightly worse on the right. The value of D-dimer of the proband was 0.89 mg/L (reference range: <0.3 mg/L). White blood cell (WBC) count was 6.2×10^9/L (reference range: $3.69\text{-}9.16\times10^9$/L) with 53.7% (reference range: 50-70%) neutrophils. CT angiography of pulmonary vessels at onset showed filling defect in lower left pulmonary artery. Contrast-enhanced CT scan of lower abdomen at onset showed right superior external iliac vein and femoral vein thrombosis.

The proband's father (I:1) who had a history of lower limb DVT, died suddenly at the age of 60, and the cause of his death was unknown. The proband's mother (I:2) died of natural causes at the age of 80. The proband's older brother (II:1) who had a history of lower limb DVT, died of cerebral infarction at the age of 37. The proband's older sister (II:3) presented with right leg swelling at the age of 58. Venous ultrasonography of lower limb at onset showed right popliteal vein and small saphenous vein thrombosis, and she was diagnosed with DVT. The proband's another older sister (II:7) presented with left lower extremity edema at the age of 56. Measurements of the upper border of the patella showed that the left thigh was 3 cm greater in circumference than the right thigh. Venous ultrasonography of lower limb revealed left lower limb deep vein thrombosis.

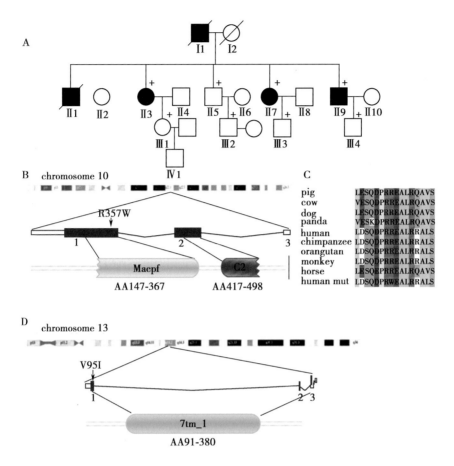

Figure 8-1-1   Pedigree and *PRF1* and *HTR2A* mutations of the VTE family.(A)The genealogical tree of VTE family. "+" indicates family members who were examined and sequenced in this study. Filled symbols indicate affected individuals. (B) The chromosomal location and genomic structure of the exons encoding the open reading frame of *PRF1*. The R357W mutation locates in the MACPF domain of protein. (C) *PRF1* orthogous conservation analysis was performed using CLUSTALW at default settings. The *PRF1* R357W mutated sequence is shown in white. (D) The chromosomal location of *HTR2A* and the location of its exons. The exon numbering indicates *HTR2A* is located on the reverse strand and the V95I mutation is location on exon 1. (International Journal Of Clinical And Experimental Medicine,2015,8(5):7951-7957)

Exon capture and next-generation sequencing

Exome sequencing was performed on 8 members of the family with VTE. Genomic DNA was extracted from peripheral blood using QIAamp DNA Blood Midi Kit and sheared by sonication. Exonic DNA was then captured using SureSelect Human All Exon 50Mb kit (Agilent Technologies). The kit contains a pool of RNA-based 120-mer capture oligomers targeting 51,646,629 bases of 213,384 consensus coding sequences and their flanking regions. The Illumina Hiseq2000 platform was applied in sequencing the exon-enriched DNA following the manufacturer's instructions.

Sequence mapping and single nucleotide variation identification

Raw sequencing reads were processed by Fastx-toolkit pipeline (http://hannonlab. cshl.edu/fastx_toolkit) to remove adapter sequences and low quality sequences. Then the reads were aligned to the human reference genome sequences, UCSC hg19 (http:// hgdownload.soe.ucsc.edu/downloads.html#human) using Burrows-Wheeler Aligner (BWA) software[10]. Sequence reads which could not be aligned to the designed target regions were filtered out and duplicate reads were further removed by SAMtools software [11]. Variations including single nucleotide variation (SNV) as well as small insertion and deletion (Indel, <10 bp) were called with the SAMtools software package. The variations should meet the following criteria: mapping quality $\geqslant 40$, SNV quality $\geqslant 20$, indel quality $\geqslant 50$ and $\geqslant 5$ reads covered. Any two or more SNVs located in a 5-bp window or SNVs overlapping with an Indel were discarded. The SNVs identified were further filtered by dbSNP 137, HapMap database (ftp://ftp.ensembl.org/pub/release-62/ variation/homo_sapiens/) and 1000 Genomes databases to remove known SNVs and the variants that remained were considered to be 'novel' SNVs. Gene transcript annotation databases (http://snp-nexus.org/index.html) were used for transcript identification and for determining amino acid changes of these 'novel' SNVs [12]. Amino acid changes were annotated according to the largest transcript of genes. PolyPhen2 (http://genetics.bwh. harvard.edu/pph2/) was applied to assess the functional impact of non-synonymous SNVs[13].

Examining PRF1, HTR2A and ABCC8 mutations in control individuals

The mutations of PRF1, HTR2A and ABCC8 were further examined in 100 ethnically matched non-related controls. Primers for both PCR amplification and Sanger sequencing were as following: CCGCTGAGCCATGGCACACA (Forward), and CGGAAGTGGTTGGCGGCCAT (Reverse) for PRF1, TGGACACGGGCATGACAAGGA (Forward), and AGCTCAACTACGAACTCCCTAATGCA (Reverse) for HTR2A and CCCCTGGGGCTGCCTACCTT (Forward), and CCCCAGACAACAGGAGCTAGG (Reverse) for ABCC8, respectively.

Examination of differentiation antigens on immune cells

2 ml of fasting venous blood was obtained from 8 members in the morning, and then the

sample was added into the ET tube. The differentiation antigens on the immune cells including CD_3, CD_4, CD_8, CD_{19} and $CD_{16}CD_{56}$ in 8 members of the VTE family (II:3, II:5, II:7, II:9, III:1, III:2, III:3 and III:4) were examined by BECKMANCOULTER EPICS XL-II flow cytometer.

Detection of complement components

Complement factors C3 and C4 levels were detected by nephelometry (BN II; Siemens, Germany). Total haemolytic complement (CH50) activity was measured by liposome immunoassay using an automated biochemistry analyser (Beckman DxC-800). This study has been approved by the Ethics Committee of Tongji University, and informed consent form was also obtained.

Exome Sequencing

Exome sequencing was performed on 3 affected individuals (II:3, II:7 and II:9) and 5 unaffected members (II:5, III:1, III:2, III:3 and III:4) in the VTE family (Figure 8-1-1A). An average of 5.5 Gb (110-folds of the target region) raw sequencing data were generated per individual, in which approximately 83% of the reads could be successfully mapped to the UCSC hg19 reference genome using the BWA short read aligner. After removing duplicated reads, approximately 3 Gb sequence data per sample were obtained and mapped to the targeted sequences with a mean coverage of 55-fold. More than 90% of the targeted sequences were sufficiently covered. A total of ~30,000 single nucleotide variants (SNVs) were detected in each sample, among which 822 to 1,355 novel SNVs were not present in dbSNP 137, 1000 Genomes or HapMap databases. Only 15 SNVs were shared by 3 affected patients (II:3, II:7 and II:9) but not by the unaffected members, among which mutations of PRF1, HTR2A, and ABCC8 were predicted to be functionally damaged to their encoded proteins based on PolyPhen 2 mutation annotation databases (Table 8-1-2). Further Sanger sequencing identified ABCC8 R298C mutation in one of 100 ethnically matched control individuals, suggesting that it is unlikely to be a pathogenic mutation of VTE.

Mutations of 2 genes predicted to be functionally damaged

PRF1 R357W mutation

PRF1 gene (perforin 1, pore forming protein) consists of 3 exons and encodes a protein of 555 amino acids. The protein is a key effector molecule for T-cell- and natural killer-cell-mediated cytolysis, capable of lysing a variety of target cells non-specifically. Figure

8-1-1B shows that the R357W mutation located in the MACPF domain of PRF1 protein also existed in the membrane attack complex proteins of complement (C6, C7, C8α, C8β and C9) [14]. To study the evolutionary conservation of the R357 residue, a CLUSTALW analysis was performed on orthogues of PRF1 of different mammal species. Figure 8-1-1C shows the results of the orthologous conservation analyses; the conclusion drawn is that the R357 residue is conserved in evolution and has never been observed to be mutated.

HTR2A V95I mutation

The HTR2A V95I is another mutation not reported in VTE. It consists of 3 exons encoding 471 amino acids and is associated with susceptibility to schizophrenia and obsessive-compulsive disorder [15]. Figure 8-1-1 D shows V95I mutation in the 7tm_1 domian of HTR2A.

Expression of differentiation antigens on immune cells and complements were detected in 8 members of the VTE family (Table 8-1-1), and it showed that the number of NK cells was decreased, the levels of CD_8, C3 and C4 were in the normal range, and the level of CH50 was significantly increased in these members.

Table 8-1-1   Expression of differentiation antigens on immune cells and complements in 8 members of the VTE family.

	II:3	II:5	II:7	II:9	III:1	III:2	III:3	III:4
Age at Examination (years)	62	59	56	50	35	30	26	21
CD_3 (60-85 %)	74.7	52↓	76.3	78.6	48.7↓	56.7↓	69.3	80.1
CD_4 (24.5-48.8 %)	44.1	30.5	51.8↑	45.3	27.3	23.4↓	35.7	30.7
CD_8 (18.5-42.1 %)	23.4	18.6	20.8	31.8	18.0↓	26.1	29.7	35.3
CD_4/CD_8 (1.02-1.94 %)	1.88	1.6	2.49↑	1.42	1.52	0.9↓	1.2	0.87↓
$NKCD_{16}CD_{56}$ (8.6~21.1 %)	5.32↓	23.2↑	7.13↓	7.54↓	42.8↑	25.9↑	15.7	15.0
CD_{19} (8~20 %)	11.4	16.9	6.35↓	10.0	8.1	1.9	8.3	6.16↓
CH50 (23-46U/ml)	48↑	—	42	49.6↑	38	—	—	50↑
C3(0.9-1.8g/L)	0.99	1.19	0.92	1.2	1.03	1.52	1.05	1.69
C4(0.1-0.4g/L)	0.26	0.26	0.23	0.26	0.18	0.31	0.21	0.32

" ↑ " indicates the level was higher than the upper limit of the normal range. " ↓ " indicates the level was less than the lower limit of the normal range.

Exome sequencing method has been used to find a causal gene underlying rare Mendelian disorders [16]. In the present study, we showed the sequencing of the exome of 8 members from a four-generation Han Chinese family with VTE. Among 3 affected individuals, mutations of PRF1 gene located in chromosome 10 and HTR2A gene located in chromosome 13 were predicted to be functionally damaged to their encoded proteins.

The R357W mutation of PRF1 gene and the V95I mutation of HTR2A were detected in the 3 affected members but not in the 5 normal members of the family (II:5, III:1, III:2, III:3 and III:4) or in 100 normal controls, indicating that VTE has a genetic component. (Table 8-1-2).

Table 8-1-2   List of mutations in 3 genes predicted to be damaging shared by 3 affected individuals.

Chr	Site	Ref	Mut	Gene	II3[a]	II5[b]	II7[a]	II9[a]	III1[b]	III2[b]	III3[b]	III4[b]
chr10	72358408	G	A	PRF1	Y[c]	N	Y	Y	N	N	N	N
chr13	47469759	C	T	HTR2A	Y	N	Y	Y	N	N	N	N
chr11	17482154	G	A	ABCC8	Y	N	Y	Y	Y	N	N	N

a. Patients in the VTE family
b. Controls in the VTE family
c. "Y" means the individual carries the amino acid alteration, and "N" means does not.

Smeeth et al. reported that the risk of VTE significantly increased after acute infection, and infection might be the trigger of VTE [17]. However, it is important to note that VTE occurs in only some of the patients who were infected, not most of them. Therefore, under what conditions, infection can trigger the occurrence of VTE?

The R357W mutation was identified in MACPF (MAC component/perforin) domain of PRF1 protein. MACPF domain exists both in the perforin secreted by cytotoxic T lymphocytes and NK cells and in the MAC of complement (C6-C9) [18-20]. The R357W mutation of PRF1 indicates that the structures of NK cells, CD_8 T cells and MAC may be abnormal, which may cause impaired capability of killing infected or tumor cells. We have reported that the mRNA expression of granzyme secreted by T cells was significantly down-regulated in symptomatic VTE patients, as compared to the control group [21], which suggests that the capability of killing infected or tumor cells is impaired in CD_8 T cells. The steps of killing alloantigen by NK cells, CD_8T cells and the membrane attack complex include membrane perforation and release of the granzyme, either of which if abnormal can lead to immune dysfunction. The R357W mutation identified in this report is consistent with the result that the mRNA expression of granzyme was significantly down-regulated in symptomatic VTE patients. These results are a manifestation of a decrease in different aspects of killing heterotypic cells, leading to decreased immune function.

Acute venous thrombosis is mainly red thrombus which is susceptible to being broken down and autolyzing. In acute venous thrombosis, delayed thrombolysis and guiding-catheter thrombectomy are often effective, which may be ascribed to the fact that the thrombus is mainly composed of fibrinogens [3]. In our previous studies, tandem mass spectrometry was performed to analyze the red thrombus in acute PE, and showed the core protein of this red thrombus was integrin β1, β2 and β3. Furthermore, immunohistochemistry confirmed that the dark brown integrins β1, β2 and β3 were mainly localized on the lymphocytes, white blood cells and platelets within the thrombus. The integrins β2 and β3 on the white blood cells and platelets can bind to fibrinogens, forming filament-like network. When the network is filled with blood cells (mainly red cells), red thrombus forms [22]. The integrin β2 on the white blood cells as shown in immunohistochemistry can bind to factor X, and factor Xa is widely distributed in the fibrinogens/fibrins of filament-like network [22], suggesting that the activation of immune cells and inflammatory adherence participate in the whole process of thrombosis in VTE [22].

When the immune function is compromised, heterologous antigens can not be eliminated effectively. The integrin β2 and β3 receptors of neutrophils and platelets are activated directly or indirectly through the heterologous antigens. When the immune function is normal, heterologous antigens can be eliminated. Thus, VTE will not occur if the integrin β1, β2 and β3 receptors can not be activated. Therefore, immune function is the intrinsic condition for the occurrence of VTE.

In this report, the level of CH50 in 3 VTE patients was elevated, indicating acute inflammation reaction in VTE patients. Decreased NK cell function is associated with the occurrence of VTE, however, it is difficult to connect it with the mutation of the perforin. In this report, we analyzed the mutations of immune related genes in familial VTE, providing new insights into the pathogenesis of familial VTE.

HTR2A, which encodes one of the receptors for 5-HT, consists of 3 exons encoding 471 amino acids. Approximately 90% of the human body's 5-HT is produced and distributed in enterochromaffin cells [23]. When 5-HT is released into the blood flow, it is rapidly taken up by platelets and stored in the dense granules [24], which constitute about 8% of the total 5-HT. It has been reported that serotonin 5-HT2A receptor blockers can increase risk of VTE, but the underlying mechanism is unknown [25]. In this study, the V95I mutation of HTR2A may lead to changes in the encoded protein. Therefore, we speculate that when serotonin cannot combine with its receptors effectively, the effects of serotonin 5-HT2A receptor blockers in VTE may be produced, leading to thrombus formation.

In this study, 8 members of the Chinese Han family with VTE were evaluated by exome sequencing. An 18-month follow-up study of the 8 members found that no VTE events occurred in the 5 unaffected members, and no recurrent VTE occurred in the 3 affected members who have been taking warfarin. The present study suggests that VTE patients with immunodeficiency under control of heredity should receive life-long anticoagulation for preventing VTE recurrence.

In this report, the mutations of immune related genes in familial VTE might provide new understanding of the pathogenesis of familial VTE.

(published: Int J Clin Exp Med 2015;8:7951-7).

References

1. Kahn SR, Lim W, Dunn AS, Cushman M, Dentali F, Akl EA, et al. Prevention of VTE in nonsurgical patients: Antithrombotic Therapy and Prevention of Thrombosis, 9th ed: American College of Chest Physicians Evidence-Based Clinical Practice Guidelines. Chest. 2012;141(2 Suppl):e195S-226S.

2. Zoller B, Ohlsson H, Sundquist J, Sundquist K. Familial risk of venous thromboembolism in first-, second- and third-degree relatives: a nationwide family study in Sweden. Thrombosis and haemostasis. 2013;109(3):458-63.

3. Reitsma PH. Genetic heterogeneity in hereditary thrombophilia. Haemostasis. 2000;30 Suppl 2:1-10.

4. Duan Q, Gong Z, Song H, Wang L, Yang F, Lv W, et al. Symptomatic venous thromboembolism is a disease related to infection and immune dysfunction. International journal of medical sciences. 2012;9(6):453-61.

5. Wang L, Zhang X, Duan Q, Lv W, Gong Z, Xie Y, et al. Rod-like bacteria and recurrent venous thromboembolism. American journal of respiratory and critical care medicine. 2012;186(7):696.

6. Wang L, Gong Z, Liang A, Xie Y, Liu SL, Yu Z, et al. Compromised T-cell immunity and virus-like structure in a patient with pulmonary hypertension. American journal of respiratory and critical care medicine. 2010;182(3):434-5.

7. Wang L, Song H, Gong Z, Duan Q, Liang A. Acute pulmonary embolism and dysfunction of CD3 CD8 T cell immunity. American journal of respiratory and critical care medicine. 2011;184(11):1315.

8. Haoming S, Lemin W, Zhu G, Aibin L, Yuan X, Wei L, et al. T cell-mediated immune deficiency or compromise in patients with CTEPH. American journal of respiratory and critical care medicine. 2011;183(3):417-8.

9. Xiang-Hua Y, Le-Min W, Ai-Bin L, Zhu G, Riquan L, Xu-You Z, et al. Severe acute respiratory syndrome and venous thromboembolism in multiple organs. American journal of respiratory and critical care medicine. 2010;182(3):436-7.

10. Li H, Durbin R. Fast and accurate short read alignment with Burrows-Wheeler transform. Bioinformatics. 2009;25(14):1754-60.

11. Li H, Handsaker B, Wysoker A, Fennell T, Ruan J, Homer N, et al. The sequence alignment/map format and SAMtools. Bioinformatics. 2009;25(16):2078-9.

12. Dayem Ullah AZ, Lemoine NR, Chelala C. SNPnexus: a web server for functional annotation of novel and publicly known genetic variants (2012 update). Nucleic acids research. 2012;40(Web Server issue):W65-70.

13. Adzhubei IA, Schmidt S, Peshkin L, Ramensky VE, Gerasimova A, Bork P, et al. A method and server for predicting damaging missense mutations. Nature methods. 2010;7(4):248-9.

14. Peitsch MC, Tschopp J. Assembly of macromolecular pores by immune defense systems. Current opinion in cell biology. 1991;3(4):710-6.

15. Nicolini H, Arnold P, Nestadt G, Lanzagorta N, Kennedy JL. Overview of genetics and obsessive-compulsive disorder. Psychiatry research. 2009;170(1):7-14.

16. Ng SB, Buckingham KJ, Lee C, Bigham AW, Tabor HK, Dent KM, et al. Exome sequencing identifies the cause of a mendelian disorder. Nature genetics. 2010;42(1):30-5.

17. Smeeth L, Cook C, Thomas S, Hall AJ, Hubbard R, Vallance P. Risk of deep vein thrombosis and pulmonary

embolism after acute infection in a community setting. Lancet. 2006;367(9516):1075-9.

18. Tschopp J, Masson D, Stanley KK. Structural/functional similarity between proteins involved in complement- and cytotoxic T-lymphocyte-mediated cytolysis. Nature. 1986;322(6082):831-4.

19. Shinkai Y, Takio K, Okumura K. Homology of perforin to the ninth component of complement (C9). Nature. 1988;334(6182):525-7. Epub 1988/08/11.

20. Voskoboinik I, Smyth MJ, Trapani JA. Perforin-mediated target-cell death and immune homeostasis. Nature reviews Immunology. 2006;6(12):940-52.

21. Song HM, Gong Z, Wang LM, Zhang XY. [The expression of T cell immune-related gene mRNAs in peripheral blood mononuclear cells from patients with venous thromboembolism]. Zhonghua nei ke za zhi. 2012;51(7):551-3.

22. Wang LM, Duan QL, Yang F, Yi XH, Zeng Y, Tian HY, Lv W and Jin Y. Activation of circulated immune cells and inflammatory immune adherence are involved in the whole process of acute venous thrombosis. Int J Clin Exp Med 2014; 7: 566-572.

23. Mawe GM, Coates MD, Moses PL. Review article: intestinal serotonin signalling in irritable bowel syndrome. Alimentary pharmacology & therapeutics. 2006;23(8):1067-76.

24. Maurer-Spurej E, Pittendreigh C, Solomons K. The influence of selective serotonin reuptake inhibitors on human platelet serotonin. Thrombosis and haemostasis. 2004;91(1):119-28.

25. Wu CS, Chang CM, Chen CY, Wu EC, Wu KY, Liang HY, et al. Association between antidepressants and venous thromboembolism in Taiwan. Journal of clinical psychopharmacology. 2013;33(1):31-7.

Chapter 9

1. The patients with acute PE and Dysfunction of CD_3CD_8 T cells

A total of 33 patients with acute PE (13male and 20 female), from 20 to 88 years of age, were recruited into the present study. A history of acute upper respiratory infection was definite within 1 to 2 weeks before hospitalization in 14 patients. Those with autoimmune disease, malignancies, or treated with immunosuppressants were excluded from this study. On the next morning after final diagnosis of PE, 2ml fasting venous blood was obtained and subjected to flow cytometry (Beckman Coulter Epics XL-II, Indianapolis, IN) for determining clusters of differentiation (CD) on the surface of T cells.

Among these 33 patients with acute PE, 13 (39.4%) had decreased CD_3 level and 13 (39.4%) had decreased CD_8 level, but the CD_4/CD_8 ratio was increased in 45.5% patients.

The decreased CD_3 level suggested the compromised signal transduction function of T cells, and the decreased CD_8 level implied the compromised ability of T cells to kill viruses. In acute PE, the decreased CD_3 and CD_8 levels, and the increased CD_4/CD_8 ratio, were similar to those in CTEPH except for the extent: the CD_3 and CD_8 levels were decreased by 4/8 (50%) and 6/8 (75%), respectively, in patients with CTEPH [1]. The common causes resulting in the decrease of CD_8 level include malignancies, medication of immunosuppressants, and viral infection. However, in the present study, no patients had maliganacies or used immunosuppressants. We previously reported virus-like microorganisms in the T lymphocytes of peripheral blood of patients with CTEPH [2] and also reported VTE in multiple organs in a patient who died of SARS [3]. Smeeth and coworkers [4] reported that acute infection was related to VTE, especially in the first 2 weeks after infection. The dysfunction of CD_3CD_8T cell immunity in patients with acute PE suggests that viral infection is associated with the occurrence of VTE.

(published:Am J Respir Crit Care Med 2011;184:1315).

References

1. Haoming S, Lemin W, Zhu G, Aibin L, Yuan X, We iL , Jinfa J, Wenjun X, Yuqin S. T cell-mediated immune deficiency or compromise in patients with CTEPH.AmJRespirCritCareMed2011;183:417-418.

2. Wang L, Gong Z, Liang A, Xie Y, Liu SL, YuZ, Wang Y. Compromised T-cell immunity and virus-like structure in a patient with pulmonary hypertension.AmJRespirCritCareMed2010;182:434-435.

3. Xiang-HuaY, Le-MinW, Ai-BinL, ZhuG, RiquanL, Xu-YouZ, Wei-Wei R, Ye-Nan W. Severe acute respiratory syndrome and venous thromboembolism in multiple organs. AmJRespirCritCareMed2010;182:436-437.

4. Smeeth L, Cook C, ThomasS, HallAJ, HubbardR, VallanceP. Risk of Deep vein thrombosis and pulmonary embolism after acute infection in a community setting. Lancet2006;367:1075-1079.

2. T cell-mediated immune deficiency in patients with CTEPH

It is traditionally known that chronic thromboembolic pulmonary hypertension (CTEPH) is the extended stage of acute pulmonary embolism (PE) [1], but this view is difficult to explain the current clinical state of CTEPH. According to the results of our previous study on human genomics [2], this article aimed to detect the T cell-mediated immunity in CTEPH patients.

Eight CTEPH patients diagnosed in Department of Cardiology, Tongji Hospital of Tongji University from 2008 to 2010 were recruited, including 2 males and 6 females, with a mean age of 56±22 years (11~80 years). The diagnosis of CTEPH was based on the criteria developed by American Heart Association (AHA). Although these 8 patients were healthy before, they were diagnosed as CTEPH because of unknown reasons of exertional dyspnea. The cluster of differentiation (CD) on T-cell surface was detected using a conventional detection approach. All patients were followed up for one year.

The number of CD_3 T cells in 4 CTEPH patients was decreased while the number of CD_8 T cells in 6 CTEPH patients was also decreased. The ratio of CD_4/CD_8 in 5 CTEPH patients was elevated, and the number of CD_4 T cells in 3 CTEPH patients was also elevated. After 1-year follow up, 2 cases were lost, and 3 cases died of right heart failure among 8 patients. The NYHA function of these 3 died patients at the initial diagnosis was III - IV .

In this report, 8 CTEPH cases progressed rapidly. During three years, 3 cases died of right heart failure, with a high mortality rate. The number of CD_3 T cells in 4 CTEPH patients was decreased while the number of CD_8 T cells in 6 CTEPH patients was also decreased, with an elevated ratio of CD_4/CD_8 in 5 CTEPH patients. The number of CD_3 and CD_8 T cells was decreased while the ratio of CD_4/CD_8 was elevated in 2 patients out of these 3 patients receiving one-year follow up. CD_3 cells play critical roles in the transformation of T cell activation signals. CD_8 cells can kill cells that are infected by viruses (or other pathogens) in the cytoplasm in vivo. Immune deficiency or compromise of T cells is often caused by virus infection, cancer or immunosuppressive drugs. In this report, malignant tumors or use of immunosuppressive drugs were all excluded in these 8 patients, so the immune deficiency or compromise of T cells the most likely resulted from virus infection.

In our report, a girl was diagnosed as idiopathic CTEPH. The assembly, and release and budding of virus-like structures were detected in the cytoplasm of the peripheral T lymphocytes under electron microscope, indicating virus infection is involved in the pathogenesis of CTEPH. Infection and inflammation are related to the onset of CTEPH [3]. Infection may be one of the risk factors of thrombosis [4], and also may be a trigger resulting in thrombosis [5]. Virus infection not only causes the onset of venous thromboembolism (VTE), but may also be an important etiological factor of CTEPH. This report indicated that the function of T cells killing viruses in CTEPH patients is compromised or T cell immune deficient. Idiopathic CTEPH may be a disease of acquired T cells-medicated immune deficiency, and virus infection may be an important etiological factor of CTEPH. The author speculates that different kinds of pathogenic microorganism infections may cause different clinical types and outcomes.

(published:Am J Respir Crit Care Med 2011;183:417-8).

References

1. Alikhan R, Cohen AT, Combe S, Samama MM, Desjardins L, Eldor A, Janbon C, Leizorovicz A, Olsson CG, Turpie AG. Risk factors for venous thromboembolism in hospitalized patients with acute medical illness: Analysis of the medenox study. Arch Intern Med 2004;164:963-968.

2. Gong Z, Liang AB, Wang LM, Zhang XY, Wang Q, Huang CY, Song HM, Wang H, Shen YQ, Gao HJ, et al. [the expression and significance of immunity associated genes mrna in patients with pulmonary embolism]. Zhonghua Nei Ke Za Zhi 2009;48:666-669.

3. Pengo V, Lensing AW, Prins MH, Marchiori A, Davidson BL, Tiozzo F, Albanese P, Biasiolo A, Pegoraro C, Iliceto S, et al. Incidence of chronic thromboembolic pulmonary hypertension after pulmonary embolism. N Engl J Med 2004;350:2257-2264.

4. Quarck R, Nawrot T, Meyns B, Delcroix M. C-reactive protein: A new predictor of adverse outcome in pulmonary arterial hypertension. J Am Coll Cardiol 2009;53:1211-1218.

5. Smeeth L, Cook C, Thomas S, Hall AJ, Hubbard R, Vallance P. Risk of deep vein thrombosis and pulmonary embolism after acute infection in a community setting. Lancet 2006;367:1075-1079.

3. Symptomatic VTE is a disease related to infection and immune dysfunction

The American College of Chest Physicians (ACCP) has recommended the guidelines for the diagnosis and prevention of venous thromboembolism (VTE) since 1995. A total of 9 issues have been published by the end of 2012 [1], and the contents have also been continuously renewed. ACCP proposed that Trauma, surgery, old age, malignancies, pregnancy, heart failure and oral administration of contraceptives are the main risk factors of VTE and ACCP also proposed the concept of risk stratification for prophylaxis of VTE by which different managements were used for prevention from VTE in different risk patients [2,3]. The incidence of symptomatic VTE is not reduced but gradually increased, the reason of which may be related to the unclear pathogenesis of VTE [4].

In 2006, Smeeth et al reported that the occurrence of VTE was associated with infection, and VTE was frequently observed within 2 weeks after infection [5]. In 2010, we reported VTE in multiple organs of a patient who died of SARS, suggesting viral infection to be a cause of systemic VTE [6]. In addition, in 2010, we detected virus-like microorganisms in the lymphocytes of a young pulmonary hypertension patient with increased D-Dimer, which morphologically confirmed the attack of T cells by virus, and peripheral decreased CD_3 and CD_8 level also indicated that virus infection caused significantly compromised function of T cells [7]. In 2011, we reported the decreased CD_3 and CD_8 level with an increased CD_4/CD_8 ratio in a group of chronic thromboembolic pulmonary hypertension (CTEPH) patients, suggesting T cellular immune dysfunction and ratio imbalance in CTEPH patients [8]. In the present study, the whole human genome microarray and Gene Ontology (GO) analysis were employed to detect the targeting of symptomatic pulmonary embolism (PE). In addition, flow cytometry was performed to investigate the changes in immune cells in VTE patients, which aimed to validate the results from genome analysis. Based on the findings above, the relationship between immune dysfunction and clinical symptomatic VTE was analyzed. The CPR level in part of VTE inpatients was determined.

Genomic study

20 PE inpatients and 20 controls were randomly selected in Cardiology Department, Tongji Hospital of Tongji University. In the PE group, there were 11 males and 9 females, with a mean age of 70±14 years (44~89 years). There were 13 patients with acute PE and 7 with CTEPH. The pulmonary artery pressure was 50-108 mmHg in CTEPH patients. In the control group, 20 patients (11 males and 9 females) with a mean age of 72±14 years (44~91 years) were enrolled during the same period. No significant difference in age was found between PE patients and control patients ($P>0.05$). Malignancies, use of immunosuppressants or autoimmune diseases were excluded in all patients.

Cellular immunology

A total of 56 clinically proven VTE patients (34 with APE, 9 with DVT and 13 with CTEPH) aged 64±18 years (13~88 years) were recruited from Tongji Hospital, including 26 males and 30 females. The immunological parameters of these patients were all compared with the detection intervals of normal population.

The diagnostic criteria of acute PE were the same as the above and the diagnosis of DVT was based on the criteria previously reported [9]. The criteria for CTEPH developed by American AHA were used for the diagnosis of CTEPH [10]. In the present study, 13 patients had the mean pulmonary artery systolic pressure of 54-106 mmHg. Malignancies, use of immunosuppresants or autoimmune diseases were excluded in all patients. All patients were from Shanghai, China. The present study was approved by the Ethics Committee of Tongji Hospital and informed consent was obtained before study.

Genomic study

Extraction of total RNA

A total of 5 ml of venous EDTA anti-coagulated blood was obtained from patients of both groups and mononuclear cells were isolated by density gradient centrifugation. Red blood cell lysis buffer (Qiagen, Hilden, Germany) was used to isolate mononuclear cells and total RNA was extracted from mononuclear cells with TRIzol (Invitrogen, Carlsbad, USA) followed by purification with RNeasy column (QIAGEN). Treatment with DNase was performed to avoid the influence by genomic DNA. Quantification of extracted RNA was performed with Nanodrop ND-1000 spectrophotometer (Nanodrop Technology, Cambridge, UK).

Gene expression profiling

Agilent G4112A Whole Human Genome Oligo Microarrays were purchased from Agilent (USA). A microarray is composed of 44,290 spots including 41,675 genes or transcripts, 314 negative control spots, 1924 positive control spots and 359 blank spots. The functions of more than 70% of genes in the microarray have been known. All patients of both groups were subjected to microarray analysis.

Sample marking and hybridization

Indirect approach was applied to mark samples. About 1 μg of total RNA was reversely transcribed into double strand cDNA. After purification, in vitro amplification was performed with Agilent Low RNA Input Linear Amplification Kit (Agilent, Pal alto, USA) and modified UTP [aaUTP, 5-(3-aminoally1)-UTP] was used to replace UTP. The integrated aaUTP can interact with Cy3 NHS ester, forming fluorescent products, which are then used for hybridization. The integration rate of fluorescence can be determined with a NanodropND-1000 spectrophotometer. Then, hybridization mixture was prepared with Agilent oligonucleotide microarray in situ hybridization plus kit. About 750 ng of fluorescent products were fragmented at 60 ℃ and hybridization was conducted in Human Whole-Genome 60-mer oligo-chips (G4112F, Agilent Technologies) at 60℃ for 17 h at 10 rpm. After hybridization, the chips were washed with Agilent Gene Expression Wash Buffer according to manufacturer's instructions. Original signals were obtained Agilent scanner and Feature Extraction software. The standardization of original signals was carried out with RMA standardized method and standardized signal values were used for screening of differentially expressed genes.

RT-PCR

The spots in the microarray were randomly selected and their expressions were confirmed by RT-PCR. Among genes with differential expressions, 3 genes were randomly selected and these genes and house keeping gene (GAPDH) were subjected to RT-PCR. The relative expressions were expressed as the expressions of target genes normalized by that of GAPDH ($2^{-\triangle\triangle Ct}$). Melting curve and $2^{-\triangle\triangle Ct}$ method were used to compare the difference in the expressions between control group and PE group. Results from RT-PCR were consistent with microarray analysis.

Go analysis

Gene Ontology organizes gene function into hierarchical categories based on biological process, molecular function and cellular component. Fisher's exact test was applied for over representation of selected genes in GO biological categories. In order to assess the significance of a particular category by random chance, false discovery rate (FDR) was estimated for all of categories. After 5,000 re-samplings, FDR was defined as FDR=1-Nk/T, where Nk refers to the subtracted number which was from Fisher's test in random samples. We specified the threshold of significant GO as p-value<0.05, FDR<0.05 and enrichment parameters. Enrichment represents the degree of gene expression significance. The equation of enrichment is as follows

$R_e=(n_f/n)/(N_f/N)$[11], where n_f is the number of significant genes within the particular category, n is the total number of genes within the same category, N_f is the number of significant genes in the entire microarray, N is the number of all genes tested.

Significant differential gene expression analysis

Agilent Feature extraction software was used to collect original data from microarray followed by analysis with robust multichip average (RMA). Gene intensity data between PE group and control group were compared with *t* test after calibration with a stochastic variance model. Differentially expressed genes were identified from whole genomes. Independent-Samples T Test was used to compare mRNA levels in samples from PE patients and controls. Statistical tests were performed using SPSS 17.0, and p values <0.05 were considered significant. Before t test, test for equality of variances was performed, if variances were not equal, t test result would be corrected.

Detection of differentiation antigens on immune cells

Sample collection: the fasting venous blood (2 ml) was collected in the morning and added to the ET tube. Flow cytometry was performed to detect the differentiation antigens on immune cells with BECKMANCOULTER EPICS XL-II flow cytometer. In 56 patients, the CD_3, CD_4, CD_8, and CD_{19} were detected, and the NK cell marker $CD_{16}CD_{56}$ was detected in 50 patients.

CRP determination

The CRP level in VTE patients was detected by scintillation turbidimetry.

GO analysis in genomic study

GO analysis targets the compromised immune functions of T cells and the decreased expression of immune receptor complex in PE patients.

mRNA expressions of neutrophils-related genes

Among 12 genes related to the activation and chemotaxis of neutrophils, the mRNA expressions of 9 genes were significantly up-regulated in PE group (Figure 9-3-1).

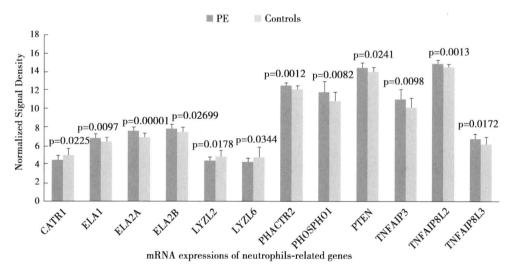

Figure 9-3-1   mRNA expressions of neutrophils-related genes (International Journal Of Medical Sciences,2012,9: 453-461)

mRNA expressions of monocytes and macrophages

In the PE patients, the mRNA expression of CD14, a mononuclear cell surface antigen, was markedly up-regulated and that of CD74, a macrophage activating factor, was also significantly up-regulated. In addition, the mRNA expressions related to Fc fragment of surface receptors (FCGR2A, FCGR2B, FCGR2C, ITGAL and SCARB1) were largely increased significantly (Figure 9-3-2).

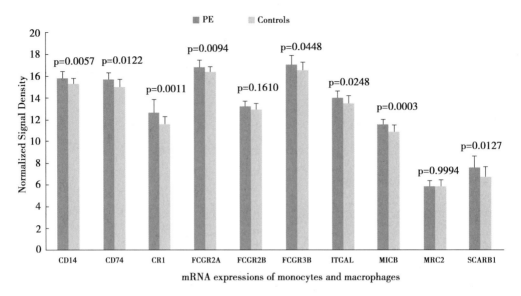

Figure 9-3-2   mRNA expressions of monocytes and macrophages (International Journal Of Medical Sciences,2012,9: 453-461)

mRNA expressions of complements related genes

The mRNA expressions of C_1 and C_3 remained unchanged. In PE group, the mRNA expressions of C_{4b}, C_5, C_{5b} as well as their receptors and complement integrins were markedly up-regulated but those of membrane attack complex component C_6, C_7, and C_9 were significantly down-regulated when compared with the control group (Figure 9-3-3).

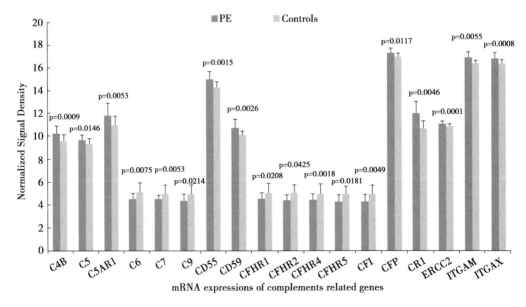

Figure 9-3-3   mRNA expressions of complements related genes (International Journal Of Medical Sciences,2012,9: 453-461)

mRNA expressions of genes related to cytokines and their regulating factors

In the PE group, the mRNA expressions of IFN regulatory factors, TNF and IL-10 were markedly up-regulated. IL-2 and IL-23A mRNA expressions were significantly down-regulated when compared with control group (Figure 9-3-4).

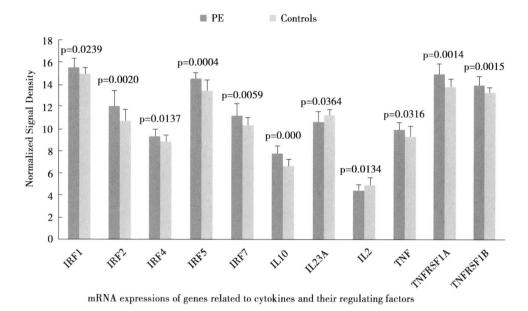

mRNA expressions of genes related to cytokines and their regulating factors

Figure 9-3-4   mRNA expressions of genes related to cytokines and their regulating factors (International Journal Of Medical Sciences,2012,9: 453-461)

mRNA expressions of NK cells related genes

In the PE group, the expression of killer lectin-like receptor (KLR) was markedly down-regulated when compared with control group, and the NCR1 mRNA expression was also markedly down-regulated (Figure 9-3-5).

mRNA expressions of B cells related genes

Only CD86 mRNA expression was significantly up-regulated in PE group (Figure 9-3-6).

mRNA expressions of T cell mediated cellular immunity

In the PE group, the mRNA expressions of T cell mediated cellular immunity, protein kinases related to transmembrane signal transduction (protein tyrosine kinase-ZAP70), T cell surface antigens (especially CD_3), membrane surface immune receptor complex and T cell granzymes were markedly down-regulated when compared with the control group (Figure 9-3-7).

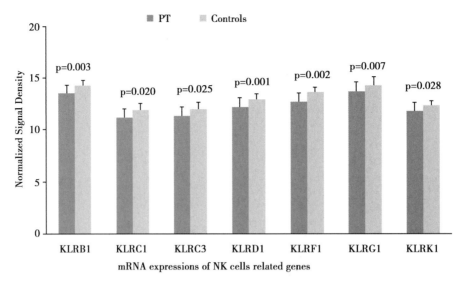

Figure 9-3-5　mRNA expressions of NK cells related genes (International Journal Of Medical Sciences,2012,9: 453-461)

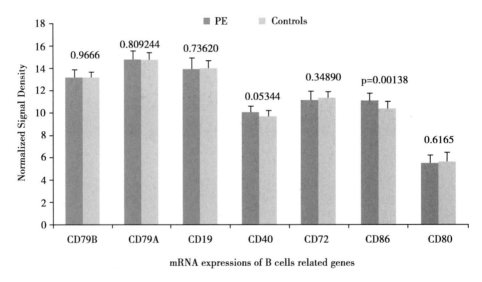

Figure 9-3-6　mRNA expressions of B cells related genes (International Journal Of Medical Sciences,2012,9: 453-461)

Findings in cellular immunology

A total of 6 parameters (CD_3, CD_4, CD_8, CD_4/CD_8, CD_{19} and $CD_{16}CD_{56}$) were measured in the 56 PE patients, and 53 had abnormalities in one or more parameters: 27 had abnormal CD_3 expression (decreased in 25 and increased in 2) (Figure 9-3-8A); 18 had aberrant CD_4 expression (decreased in 10 and increased in 8) (Figure 9-3-8B); 26 had abnormal CD_8 expression(decreased in 25 and increased in 1) (Figure 9-3-8C); 30 had aberrant CD_4/CD_8 ratio (decreased in 7 and increased in 23) (Figure 9-3-8D); 23 had

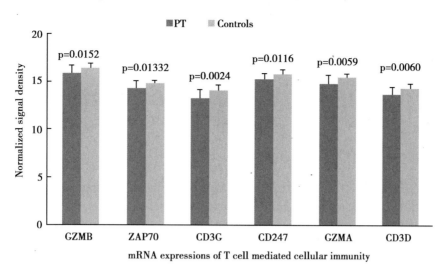

Figure 9-3-7   mRNA expressions of T cell mediated cellular immunity
(International Journal Of Medical Sciences,2012,9: 453-461)

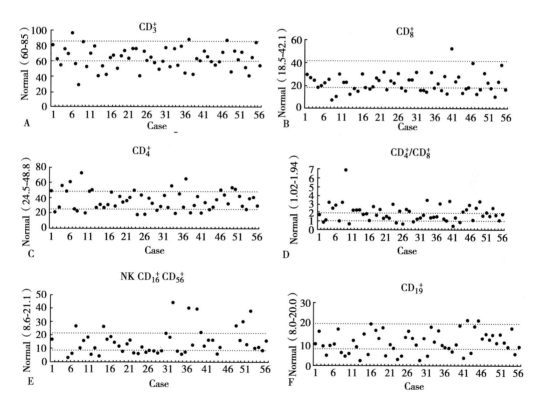

Figure 9-3-8   Findings in cellular immunology. A, 27 had abnormal CD_3 expression (decreased in 25 and increased in 2); B, 18 had aberrant CD_4 expression (decreased in 10 and increased in 8); C, 26 had abnormal CD_8 expression(decreased in 25 and increased in 1); D, 30 had aberrant CD_4/CD_8 ratio (decreased in 7 and increased in 23); E, 23 had abnormal NK $CD_{16}CD_{56}$ expression in 50 patients (decreased in 14 and increased in 9); F, 17 had aberrant CD_{19} expression in 56 patients (decreased in 15 and increased in 2)

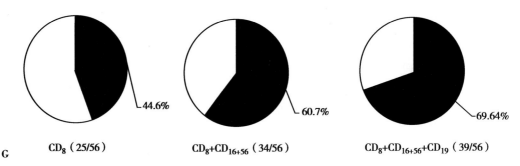

G

CD$_8$ (25/56)   CD$_8$+CD$_{16+56}$ (34/56)   CD$_8$+CD$_{16+56}$+CD$_{19}$ (39/56)

Figure 9-3-8(continued)   G, The CD$_8$ expression was decreased in 25 out of 56 patients(44.6%), the CD$_8$ and CD$_{16}$CD$_{56}$ expressions were decreased in 34 out of 56 patients(60.7%), and the CD$_8$, CD$_{16}$CD$_{56}$ and CD$_{19}$ expressions were decreased in 39 out of 56 patients(69.64%) (International Journal Of Medical Sciences,2012,9: 453-461)

abnormal NK CD$_{16}$CD$_{56}$ expression in 50 patients (decreased in 14 and increased in 9) (Figure 9-3-8E) and 17 had aberrant CD$_{19}$ expression in 56 patients (decreased in 15 and increased in 2)(Figure 9-3-8F); The CD$_8$ expression was decreased in 25 out of 56 patients(44.6%), the CD$_8$ and CD$_{16}$CD$_{56}$ expressions were decreased in 34 out of 56 patients(60.7%), and the CD$_8$, CD$_{16}$CD$_{56}$ and CD$_{19}$ expressions were decreased in 39 out of 56 patients(69.8%)(Figure 9-3-8G).

CRP determination

In 56 VTE patients, 44 patients received CRP determination. The CRP level in 35 out of 44 patients (79.5%) was higher than normal range (Figure 9-3-9).

The Go analysis of the genomic study targeted the decreased immune function of T cells and immune receptor complex in PE patients, suggesting that the occurrence of PE is closely related to the immune dysfunction. Statistical analysis revealed that the mRNA expressions of genes associated with innate immunity and cytokines were markedly up-

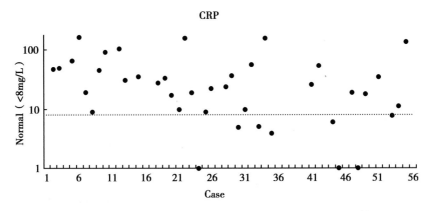

Figure 9-3-9   The CRP level in 35 out of 44 patients (79.5%) was higher than normal range (International Journal Of Medical Sciences,2012,9: 453-461)

regulated and those related to the cellular immunity of T cells and NK cells significantly down-regulated. In addition, cytological experiment indicated 6 parameters related to immune function were abnormal in 53 of 56 VTE patients. The expressions of CD_3 and CD_8 were markedly reduced and the CD_4/CD_8 ratio significantly increased. The number of $CD_{16}CD_{56}$ and CD_{19} cells was reduced. The results from cytological examination and genome analysis were consistent.

Among the 56 patients with VTE, 25 (44.6%) had decreased CD_3 T cells, 25 had reduced CD_8 T cells and 23 (41%) had increased CD_4/CD_8 ratio. These findings indicated that the ability of T cells to recognize antigen and transmit activation signals was significantly compromised, and the capability of T cells to kill the pathogen infected cells decreased. The compromised T cell immune function is often identified in patients with malignancy, use of immunosuppressant, viral infection or malnutrition [12, 13]. In the present study, none of patients had malignancies or were treated with immunosuppressants. Therefore, the pathogenesis of VTE might be closely related to viral infection or malnutrition. In our report, the synthesis and release of virus-like micro-organisms were noted in the lymphocytes under an electron microscope in a young pulmonary hypertension patient with increased D-Dimer [7].

Among 56 patients with VTE, 14 had decrease of $CD_{16}CD_{56}$ NK cells, which suggests that the ability of NK cells to kill intracellular pathogens including virus is impaired. CD_{19} is only expressed on the B lymphocytes of normal hemopoietic system and the follicular dendritic cells (FDC) of germinal center. The expression of CD_{19} is detectable back to progenitor B cells and present during the maturation of B lymphocytes. Once the B cells differentiate into plasma cells, the CD_{19} expression is absent. CD_{19} involves in the flux of Ca^{2+} in the B lymphocytes, and can regulate the activation and proliferation of B cells [14]. Among 56 VTE patients, 15 had decreased CD_{19} expression, which suggests that the activity and proliferation of B cells are compromised.

In 53 of 56 VTE patients, the expressions of CD_3, CD_8, $CD_{16}CD_{56}$ and CD_{19} were separately or combinedly down-regulated or the CD_4/CD_8 ratio was abnormal. These results imply that the occurrence of VTE is closely related to the immune function. In the present study, $CD_{16}CD_{56}$ T cells and/or CD_8 T cells were decreased in 34 out of 56 VTE patients (60.7%). Down-regulation of $CD_{16}CD_{56}$, CD_8 and/or CD_{19} was found in 39 out of 56 patients (69.64%). These findings indicate that the symptomatic VTE is associated with the decrease of innate immunity and adaptive immunity in more than 2/3 of patients. Moreover, 53 VTE patients (94.6%) had one or more immune dysfunctions.

Among the 56 VTE patients, only 3 had normal immune function. Two patients were a 31-year-old male acute PE patient and 62-year-old female acute PE patient who did not receive genetic testing. The remaining one patient was a 66-year-old female patient who was diagnosed as CTEPH and underwent splenectomy 20 years before. For patients with abnormal immune function on admission, it was difficult to confirm when the immune function became abnormal. However, we found that more than 10 patients with down-regulation of CD_8 and $CD_{16}CD_{56}$ developed symptomatic VTE sequentially.

More than 50% of the 56 VTE patients had symptoms of respiratory infection or a history of respiratory infection recently. Among the 56 VTE patients, CRP was measured in 44 of them and 35 (79.5%) had increase of CRP, which implies inflammation is related to the occurrence of VTE. In response to the invasion of foreign pathogens to human body, instantaneous innate immune response occurs within 0-4 hours after infection, and early innate immune response occurs 4-96 hours after infection [15, 16]. DVT and PE often occurred after 2-10 days postoperatively, which coincided with the infection process of innate and adaptive immune function [17].

During the 3-year follow up period, 21 VTE patients (40%; including those died) were lost to follow up. Among the patients receiving follow up, all were treated with warfarin for anti-coagulation. In addition, immunological examination and detection of D-Dimer were also carried out at designed time points. Our results showed that about 30% of VTE patients receiving follow up did not have increase of D-Dimer level any more at 0.1~1 year after warfarin discontinuation when the immunological examination and detection of D-D dimer showed normal.

Of the 56 patients with symptomatic VTE, the relationship between VTE and immune dysfunction was found in 53 (94.6%). Nevertheless, patients with immune dysfunction did not develop symptomatic VTE in a short time. The compromised or disorganized immune function may be the internal cause of susceptibility to acquired VTE, and infection acts as a triggering factor of acquired VTE. When the pathogens invade the subjects with immune dysfunction, the pathogens can not be completely removed by the immune system. Thus, patients with compromised or disorganized immune function are susceptible to acquired VTE.

(published:Int J Med Sci 2012;9:453-61).

References

1. Kahn SR, Lim W, Dunn AS, et al. Prevention of VTE in nonsurgical patients: Antithrombotic Therapy and Prevention of Thrombosis, 9th ed: American College of Chest Physicians Evidence-Based Clinical Practice Guidelines.Chest. 2012;141(2 Suppl):e195S-226S.

2. Geerts WH, Pineo GF, Heit JA, et al. Prevention of venous thromboembolism: the Seventh ACCP Conference on Antithrombotic and Thrombolytic Therapy. Chest 2004;126:338S-400S.

3. Geerts WH, Bergqvist D, Pineo GF, et al. Prevention of venous thromboembolism: American College of Chest

Physicians Evidence-Based Clinical Practice Guidelines (8th Edition). Chest 2008;133:381S-453S.

4. Shackford SR, Rogers FB, Terrien CM, Bouchard P, Ratliff J, Zubis R. A 10-year analysis of venous thromboembolism on the surgical service: the effect of practice guidelines for prophylaxis. Surgery 2008;144(1): 3-11.

5. Smeeth L, Cook C, Thomas S, et al. Risk of deep vein thrombosis and pulmonary embolism after acute infection in a community setting. Lancet 2006; 367(9516):1075-9.

6. Xiang-Hua Y, Le-Min W, Ai-Bin L, et al. Severe acute respiratory syndrome and venous thromboembolism in multiple organs. Am J Respir Crit Care Med 2010; 182:436-7.

7. Wang L, Gong Z, Liang A, et al. Compromised t-cell immunity and virus-like structure in a patient with pulmonary hypertension. Am J Respir Crit Care Med 2010; 182:434-5.

8. Haoming S, Lemin W, Zhu G, et al. T Cell-mediated Immune deficiency or compromise in patients with CTEPH. Am J Respir Crit Care Med 2011;183(3):417-8.

9. Qaseem A, Snow V, Barry P, et al. Current diagnosis of venous thromboembolism in primary care: a clinical practice guideline from the American Academy of Family Physicians and the American College of Physicians. Ann Intern Med, 2007;146(6):454-458.

10. McLaughlin VV, Archer SL, Badesch DB, et al. ACCF/AHA 2009 expert consensus document on pulmonary hypertension: a report of the American College of Cardiology Foundation Task Force on Expert Consensus Documents and the American Heart Association: developed in collaboration with the American College of Chest Physicians, American Thoracic Society, Inc., and the Pulmonary Hypertension Association. Circulation 2009;119(16):2250-2294.

11. Dupuy D, Bertin N, Hidalgo CA, et al. Genome-scale analysis of in vivo spatiotemporal promoter activity in Caenorhabditis elegans. Nat Biotechnol 2007; 25:663-8.

12. Zola H, Swart B, Banham A, et al. CD molecules 2006—human cell differentiation molecules. J Immunol Methods 2007; 318 (1-2): 1-5.

13. Robertson P, Scadden DT. Immune reconstitution in HIV infection and its relationship to cancer. Hematol Oncol Clin North Am 2003;17(3):703-16

14. Depoil D, Fleire S, Treanor BL, et al. CD_{19} is essential for B cell activation by promoting B cell receptor-antigen microcluster formation in response to membrane-bound ligand. Nat Immunol 2008; 9(1):63-72.

15. Zacho J, Tybjærg-Hansen A, Nordestgaard BG. C-reactive protein and risk of venous thromboembolism in the general population. Arterioscler Thromb Vasc Biol 2010;30(8):1672-8

16. Tollrian R, Harvell CD. The evolution of inducible defenses: Current ideas. In: The Ecology and Evolution of Inducible Defenses (Tollrian, R., and Harvell, CD, eds.), 1999; 306-321.

17. Cracowskia JL, Bossona JL, Baloula F, et al. Early development of deep-vein thrombosis following hip fracture surgery: the role of venous wall thickening detected by B-mode ultrasonography. Vascular Medicine 1998; 3: 269-274

4. Acute VTE and high expression of CH50

Smeeth et al. reported that the occurrence of acute venous thromboembolism (VTE) was associated with infection, particularly in the post-infection 2 weeks [1]. We have found compromised NK cell function in patients with acute pulmonary embolism (PE) [2], and immune function compromise /disorder of CD_3 and CD_8 T cells in patients with acute PE and chronic thromboembolic pulmonary hypertension (CTEPH) [3,4], indicating innate and adaptive immunity are both involved in the onset of VTE.

Complements are core molecules in the innate immune system, involved in both innate and adaptive immunity. Complements consist of 9 components, which together with factors associated with complement activity and its regulation are termed complement system. The activation of the complement system renders cascade reaction. The common end of the activation pathway forms membrane attack complex (MAC), which exerts cytolytic effect. The complement system contains 30 kinds of proteins, but not all of them are detected routinely in clinical practice. We detected the CRP, CH50, C3 and C4 levels in acute VTE patients and reported as follows.

There were 45 acute VTE patients including 22 males and 23 females, with a mean age 67.9 ± 15.2 years. The CRP level increased in 31/45 patients and remained normal in 14/45 patients. The CH50 level increased in 38/45 patients and remained normal in 7/45 patients. The C3 level decreased in 3/45 patients, increased in 2/45 patients, and remained normal in 40/45 patients. The C4 level increased in 4/45 patients and remained normal in 40/45 patients.

CRP, C3 and C4 are positive acute phase proteins. CRP is synthesized in the liver while wound or inflammation causes tissue damage. It is increased within 6-8 hours after infection, peaked within 24-48 hours. CRP can activate complement, and complement activation is an important event in inflammatory responses. CH50 reflects the activities of C1-C9 via the classic pathway, which needs the adaptive immunity after the pathogens are recognized by the antibodies. Here we report increased CH50 and CRP levels, indicting acute inflammatory reaction state. C3 and C4 protein levels in VTE patients had no significant change, while CH50 level was increased and sensitized in acute VTE patients.

(published:Int J Clin Exp Med 2014;7(8):2351-2354)

References

1. Smeeth L, Cook C, Thomas S, et al. Risk of deep vein thrombosis and pulmonary embolism after acute infection in a community setting. Lancet 2006; 367:1075-9.

2. Duan Q, Gong Z, Song H, Wang L, Yang F, Lv W, Song Y. Symptomatic venous thromboembolism is a disease related to infection and immune dysfunction. Int J Med Sci. 2012;9(6):453-61

3. Wang L, Song H, Gong Z, Duan Q, Liang A. Acute pulmonary embolism and dysfunction of CD_3 CD_8 T cell immunity. Am J Respir Crit Care Med. 2011;184:1315.

4. Haoming S, Lemin W, Zhu G, Aibin L, Yuan X, Wei L, Jinfa J, Wenjun X, Yuqin S. T cell-mediated immune deficiency or compromise in patients with CTEPH. Am J Respir Crit Care Med. 2011;183:417-8.

Part II
Arterial thrombus

Chapter 10

New viewpoints on the pathogenesis of acute arterial thrombosis

Acute myocardial infarction (AMI) is a typical arterial thrombotic event. Acute arterial thrombosis is a common disease with high morbidity worldwide.[1] Thus, arterial thrombosis has been a social burden and the consequent high morbidity and disability have been a worldwide health problem.[2] The typical pathology of acute arterial thrombosis is the rupture of soft plaque cap in the arterial endarterium, aggregation of platelets at the site of rupture and subsequent thrombosis.[3] Acute rupture of soft plaque cap has been regarded as an initiator of arterial thrombosis.[4] Some investigators speculate that soft plaques are landmines, but what events may trigger the landmine and when the landmine would be triggered are still unclear.[5] The pathogenesis is generally ascribed to the damage of vascular endothelial cells, change in blood flow and increase in the blood coagulability.[6] The rupture of instable atherosclerotic plaques and the subsequent adhesion and aggregation of platelets at the sites of rupture may trigger the thrombosis.[7] Evidence-based medicine shows atherosclerosis is closely related to multiple risk factors such as hypertension, hyperlipidemia, hyperglycemia, obesity and smoking.[8] However, the clinical phenomenon that acute arterial thrombosis also occurs in population which is not exposed to these risk factors is difficult to explain. Thus, there might be mechanisms other than the above mentioned factors involved in the pathogenesis of arterial thrombosis.

Human genomics has the advantages of wholeness, comprehensiveness and directivity. Although there is difference in the gene-guided protein synthesis among individual proteins which requires to be validated by proteomic and cytological studies, comparisons of gene expression patterns among different groups and functional analysis of differentially expressed genes may provide a general view and a new horizon for the understanding of mechanisms underlying the pathogenesis of diseases. This is a unique feature of genomics.[9,10] In our study, gene expression profiles were compared among patients with AMI (Group A), patients with stable angina (Group B) and healthy controls (Group C). Our findings may provide a new understanding on the pathogenesis of acute arterial thrombosis.

Sample clustering analysis of genes indicated that patients in Group A had a special gene expression pattern [11]. Hierarchical clustering analysis classified genes into several co-expression modules, which displayed the difference in the gene expression pattern among Group A, B and C. Functional analysis of differentially expressed genes showed that the genes with significantly down-regulated expression in Group A were related to mitochondrial metabolism, ion metabolism, activation of intracellular bilirubin, regulation of T lymphocyte activity, electron transport chain, MHC II receptor activity, regulation of lymphocyte proliferation and transcription. Genes with markedly up-regulated expression in Group A were associated with apoptosis, inflammatory response, functions of macrophages, neutrophil-mediated immune reaction, cell metabolism, cell repair, development of immune system and signaling pathways related to steroid receptors. However, the gene expression patterns were comparable between Groups B and C, suggesting the stability of biological metabolism in both groups. Besides the comparisons of gene expression patterns, the differentially expressed genes related to innate immunity and adaptive immunity were also compared among Groups A, B and C, and these genes were related to phagocytes (neutrophils and monocytes) [12], NK cells,[13] complement system, cytokines, adhesion molecules, T cells, B cells, coagulation and anti-coagulation system and fibrinolysis system. Results showed hyperfunction of phagocytes in Group A, reduced killing effect of NK cells, reduced complement-mediated membrane lysis ability, increase/decrease in IFN, interleukine (IL), and chemokines. Increase in TNF activity demonstrated the significant imbalance among cytokines. The functions of adhesion molecules were increased, and functions of CD_3 were reduced. Significant imbalance of CD_4 T cell function, a shift towards Th1 dominance, reduced killing effect of CD_8T cells and disordered B cell function were also observed. In Groups A and B, the mRNA expressions of some genes related to coagulation factors were up-regulated significantly, the mRNA expressions of genes related to several anti-coagulation factors in Group A were significantly higher than those in Groups B and C. In Groups A and B, the mRNA expressions of plasminogen activator inhibitor-1 and urokinase-type plasminogen activator were significantly up-regulated. These findings suggest that the functions of some coagulation factors and anti-coagulation factors were increased and there was a functional imbalance in the fibrinolytic system.

The immune system generally acts to defend pathogenic microorganisms. Precisely, immune system mainly functions to timely recognize and remove exogenous microbes (such as virus and bacterium) and endogenous malignant cells.[14] The immune function can be divided into innate immunity and adaptive immunity. The innate and adaptive immunity may act synergistically to clear cells with foreign and /or pathological antigens, avoiding the occurrence of diseases. The abnormal immune function may

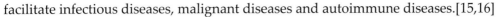

facilitate infectious diseases, malignant diseases and autoimmune diseases.[15,16]

Participants of innate immunity include phagocytes, NK cells, complement system, and cytokines, and those of adaptive immunity include T cells and B cells. Innate immunity functions can kill the exogenous pathogenic microbes (such as virus and bacterium), which is not specific for a pathogen. Cells of innate immunity may collect information of pathogens and integrate and transmit this information to adaptive immunity. Then, innate immunity and adaptive immunity interact and function synergistically to remove exogenous pathogenic microbes and endogenous malignant cells.[17,18] NK cells and CD_8T cells target the cells infected by viruses or bacteria or malignant cells, and bind to these cells via adhesion molecules. Then, both NK and CD_8 T cells release perforins and granzymes to kill the abnormal cells. [19,20] The complement system is also involved in the innate immunity and adaptive immunity. It may kill pathogenic microbes via membrane attack complex [21]. B cells mediate humeral immune response mainly through generating specific antibodies [22]. Neutrophils are involved in inflammatory reactions, can release reactive oxygen species, and phagocytize and clear pathogens.[23]

Results of human genomics exhibited a set of images presented by significantly differentially expressed genes. There is systemic immune cell balancing function collapse in acute arterial thrombotic patients. Under this situation, immune cells cannot clear exogenous pathogenic microorganisms or endogenous malignant cells timely and effectively. However, objectives with malignancies enrolled in this study were excluded, indicating that the occurrence of acute arterial thrombotic events has a close relation with stayed pathogenic microorganisms which have not been eliminated timely and effectively. And this causes consequent occurrence of arterial intima inflammation. Significantly decreased activities of MHCII receptors in A group strongly sugessted that pathogen was bacteria-like microorganism. The life time of neutrophils is 1-3 days, rupture of which could release plentiful active oxygen, causing undifferentiated damages to surrounding tissues, including damages to arterial intima cells, at the same time of killing bacteria-like microorganism. After inflammatory injuries to intima (erosive damages and rupture of soft plaque caps), adhesion and aggregation of platelets cause formation of white thrombus, which is a repair form after inflammatory repair as well as a consequence of middle and lower stages in arterial thrombotic events. Pathogenic microorganisms and their produced toxins can damage surrounding cells also. Chemotactic, aggregated and adhesive neutrophils to arterial intima cells release active oxygen, which might be the culprit causing arterial intima injuries (Figure 10-1-1,2,3,4). Psychological and mental stress situation may promote inhibition of immune system functions [24]. Sympathetic nerves increase oxidative stress on vessel wall as well as instability of artery atherosclerotic plaque [25]. Besides, results of these serial studies show that immune cell function stay in a stable imbalanced situation, while expressions

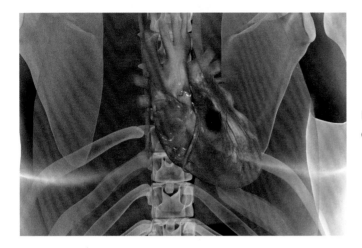

Figure 10-1-1   A simulated diagram of acute myocardial infarction

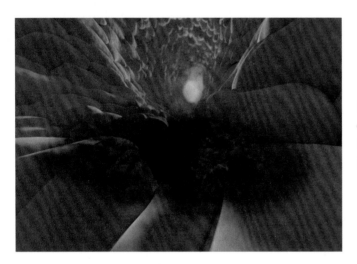

Figure 10-1-2   A simulated diagram of active substances released by leukocytes causing acute artery intima injury

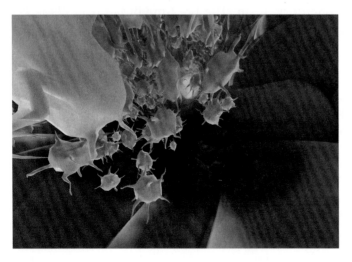

Figure 10-1-3   A simulated diagram of adhesion and aggregation of platelets at an acute artery intima injured part and a formation of white thrombus

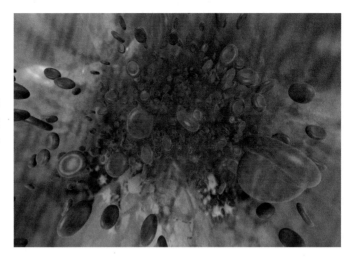

Figure 10-1-4 A simulated diagram of blood cells being involved in extension of white thrombus

of some inflammatory factors significantly increased or decreased in stable coronary disease group, indicating that patients with stable coronary diseases are in a situation of low-grade inflammatory response.

Results of this series of researches showed that mRNA expressions of some inflammatory factors related genes were upregulated or downregulated significantly in patients with stable angina pectoris, suggesting that patients with stable angina pectoris are in a status of low-grade inflammation, while mRNA expressions of genes related to immune cells indicate that immune functions stay in a relatively steady state in general.

Through comparison of mRNA expressions of genes related to the immune system (Chapter 13) and comparison at an immune cytological level, this series of researches showed that the tendency of mRNA expressions of genes related to immune cells was consistent with that of immune cell counts in AMI patients, suggesting a significantly decreased imbalance and a systemic immune cell balancing function collapse in AMI patients. Subjects with malignant tumors were excluded from this study, indicting that genesis of AMI may be related to pathogenic microorganism infections under a condition of immune cell balancing function collapse.

Through comparison of mRNA expressions of genes related to immune cells and comparison at an immune cytological level, this series of researches showed that reduction in mRNA expressions of genes related to immune cells was different from that in immune cell counts in patients with stable angina pectoris. Proteins in complement system elevated significantly, counts of NK cells, CD_3 T cells, CD_8 T cell, and CD_{19} cells decreased significantly, while mRNA expressions of genes related to immune cells stay in a relatively steady state.

Results of immunocytology and immune genomics indicate that the occurrence of AMI and SAP was related to immune cell balancing functions. AMI occurred in a condition of significant disturbance of immune cell functions and significantly decreased immune genomics expression, which is also a situation of immune cell balancing function collapse, while SAP occurred in a condition of significant disturbance of immune cell functions and relatively stable immune genomics expression. Clinical immune cell counts expressed the functional status of immune cells, while mRNA expressions of immune genomics reflected a potential compensatory function state of immune cells.

(published: Journal of Geriatric Cardiology (2015) 12: 204-207)

References

1. Yeh RW, Go AS.Rethinking the epidemiology of acute myocardial infarction: challenges and opportunities.Arch Intern Med. 2010;170(9):759-64.

2. Krumholz HM, Normand SL.Public reporting of 30-day mortality for patients hospitalized with acute myocardial infarction and heart failure. Circulation. 2008 ;118(13):1394-7.

3. Siddiqui TI, Kumar K S A, Dikshit DK.Platelets and atherothrombosis: causes, targets and treatments for thrombosis.Curr Med Chem.2013;20(22):2779-97.

4. Santos-Gallego CG, Picatoste B, Badimón JJ.Pathophysiology of acute coronary syndrome.Curr Atheroscler Rep.2014 ;16(4):401.

5. Corti R, Farkouh ME, Badimon JJ. The vulnerable plaque and acute coronary syndromes.Am J Med. 2002 Dec 1;113(8):668-80.

6. Kashyap VS, Reil TD, Moore WS, Hoang TX, Gelabert HA, Byrns RE, Ignarro LJ, Freischlag JA. Acute arterial thrombosis causes endothelial dysfunction: a new paradigm for thrombolytic therapy.J Vasc Surg. 2001;34(2):323-9.

7. Siegel-Axel DI, Gawaz M.Platelets and endothelial cells.Semin Thromb Hemost.2007 ;33(2):128-35.

8. Leone A.Relationship between cigarette smoking and other coronary risk factors in atherosclerosis: risk of cardiovascular disease and preventive measures. Curr Pharm Des.2003;9(29):2417-23.

9. Brockman JA, Tamminga CA.The human genome: microarray expression analysis.Am J Psychiatry. 2001 Aug;158(8):1199.

10. Do JH, Choi DK.Clustering approaches to identifying gene expression patterns from DNA microarray data.Mol Cells.2008 Apr 30;25(2):279-88. Epub 2008 Mar 31.

11. Wen-Wen YAN, Kun-Shan ZHANG, Qiang-Lin DUAN, Le-Min WANG Significantly reduced function of T cells in patients with acute arterialthrombosis Journal of Geriatric Cardiology (2015) 12: 287-293

12. Chuan-Rong LI, Le-Min WANG, Zhu GONG, Jin-Fa JIANG, Qiang-Lin DUAN, Wen-Wen YAN, Xiao-Hui LIU Expression characteristics of neutrophil and mononuclear-phagocyte relatedgenes mRNA in the stable angina pectoris and acute myocardial infarctionstages of coronary artery disease Journal of Geriatric Cardiology (2015) 12: 279-286

13. Wenwen Yan, Lemin Wang, Qianglin Duan, Wenjun Xu, Chuanrong Li, Feifei Huang, Yu Tang and Yongyan Chai. mRNA Expression of Inhibitory and Activating Natural Killer Cell Receptors in Patients with Acute Myocardial

Infarction and Stable Angina Pectoris. Exp Clin Cardiol. 2014;20(1):2982-2992.

14. Janeway CA, Jr, Travers P, Walport M, Shlomchik MJ. Immunobiology. 5th ed. New York: Garland Science; 2001.

15. Bansal AS, Bradley AS, Bishop KN, Kiani-Alikhan S, Ford B.Chronic fatigue syndrome, the immune system and viral infection. Brain Behav Immun. 2012 Jan;26(1):24-31. doi: 10.1016/j.bbi.2011.06.016. Epub 2011 Jul 2.

16. Ohm JE, Carbone DP.Immune dysfunction in cancer patients.Oncology (Williston Park).2002 Jan;16(1 Suppl 1):11-8.

17. Bikard D, Marraffini LA.Innate and adaptive immunity in bacteria: mechanisms of programmed genetic variation to fight bacteriophages.Curr Opin Immunol. 2012 Feb;24(1):15-20.

18. Elliott DE, Siddique SS, Weinstock JV. Innate immunity in disease.Clin Gastroenterol Hepatol.2014 May;12(5):749-55. doi: 10.1016/j.cgh.2014.03.007. Epub 2014 Mar 12.

19. Mace EM, Dongre P, Hsu HT, Sinha P, James AM, Mann SS, Forbes LR, Watkin LB, Orange JS.Cell biological steps and checkpoints in accessing NK cell cytotoxicity.Immunol Cell Biol. 2014 Mar;92(3):245-55. doi: 10.1038/icb.2013.96. Epub 2014 Jan 21.

20. Christensen ME, Waterhouse NJ.Mechanisms of CTL cytotoxicity. A reactive response to granzyme B.Immunol Cell Biol. 2010 Jul;88(5):500-1. doi: 10.1038/icb.2010.23. Epub 2010 Mar 16.

21. Ricklin D, Hajishengallis G, Yang K, Lambris JD.Complement: a key system for immune surveillance and homeostasis.Nat Immunol.2010 Sep;11(9):785-97.

22. Martin F, Chan AC.B cell immunobiology in disease: evolving concepts from the clinic.Annu Rev Immunol. 2006;24:467-96.

23. Kobayashi SD, DeLeo FR.Role of neutrophils in innate immunity: a systems biology-level approach.Wiley Interdiscip Rev Syst Biol Med. 2009 Nov-Dec;1(3):309-33.

24. JonathanP. Godbout, Ronald Glaser Stress-Induced Immune Dysregulation: Implications for Wound Healing, Infectious Disease and Cancer J NEUROIMMUNE PHARM , vol. 1, no. 4, pp. 421-427, 2006

25. Custodis F,Schirmer SH,Baumhäkel M,Heusch G,Böhm M,Laufs U Vascular pathophysiology in response to increased heart rate.J Am Coll Cardiol 2010 Dec 7;56(24):1973-83

Chapter 11

Human genomics in patients with acute myocardial infarction — pandect

Acute arterial thrombosis and differentially expressed genes— Significantly reduced function of T cells

Cardiovascular diseases (CVDs), with high morbidity, are prevalent worldwide. Atherosclerosis has been regarded as a major cause of acute arterial thrombosis (AAT). The pathogenesis of AAT has been ascribed to the injury of vascular endothelial cells, the change of blood flow and the increased blood coagulation.[1,2] AAT is the results of rupture of soft plaque cap, adhesion and aggregation of platelets at the site of rupture and then subsequent cascade of thrombosis.[3] In the present study, human genome-wide expression microarray assay was performed to investigate the mRNA expression characteristics of genes related to peripheral blood mononuclear cells (PBMC) in acute myocardial infarction (AMI) patients, stable angina pectoris (SAP) patients and healthy controls. The assay was introduced to systematically analyze the differentially expressed genes among three groups. We aimed to evaluate the intrinsic factors related to the pathogenesis of AAT according to the differences in the expressions of functional genes.

Patient information

This prospective study included three groups of subjects, 20 with AMI, 20 with SA, and 20 healthy volunteers. The baseline demographic data were displayed in Table11- 1. The AMI patients were admitted <12 hours from the onset of symptoms to our coronary care unit between January and June 2013, including 18 males and 2 females, with an average age of 58±12 (mean ± s.d.) years. All the AMI subjects were diagnosed on the basis of the following criteria: detection of a rise of cardiac biomarker values [preferably cardiac troponin] with at least one value above the 99th percentile upper reference limit and with at least one of the following: 1) symptoms of ischemia; 2) new or presumed new significant ST-segment-T wave changes or new left bundle branch block; 3) development of pathological Q waves in the ECG; 4) imaging evidence of new loss of viable myocardium or new regional wall motion abnormality; or 5) identification of an intracoronary thrombus by angiography. [4].

As the SAP group, we studied 20 patients (18 male,2 female, mean age 64±10) with exclusively effort-related angina, with a positive exercise stress test and at least one coronary stenosis detected at angiography (>70% reduction of lumen diameter). There were no significant differences between AMI and SAP patients in age, gender, smoking status, BMI, systolic blood pressure, diastolic blood pressure, LDL-C, HDL-C, triglycerides, fasting glucose or creatinine (Table11-1-1).

Table 11-1-1   Baseline demographic data in three groups (mean ± s.d.)

	AMI(a) (N=20)	SAP (b) (N=20)	Con(c) (N=20)	P (all)	P (a v b)
Age(years)	57.8±11.9	63.6±9.9	28.8±3.3	0.000	0.251
Sex(M/F)	18/2	18/2	17/3	0.853	1.0
BMI(kg/m^2)	23.6±2.6	22.8±2.7	21.3±1.8	0.102	0.56
Smoke(NO./d)	13.6±12.2	9.8±10.3	0	0.00	0.648
Syst(mmHg)	128.6±15.3	123.0±12.1	120.8±7.2	0.115	0.501
Diast(mmHg)	67.0±8.0	73.0±8.0	71.6±3.2	0.017	0.064
LDL-C(mmol/L)	2.5±1.0	2.1±0.8	2.9±0.5	0.327	0.548
Triglycerides(mmol/L)	1.6±1.1	1.5±1.4	1.2±0.4	0.73	0.762
HDL-C(mmol/L)	0.8±0.7	0.9±0.2	1.3±0.2	0.000	0.803
FPG(mmol/L)	5.4±0.9	5.0±0.8	4.9±0.5	0.61	0.082
Scr(umol/L)	87.2±19.6	76.9±14.8	72.2±6.4	0.327	0.138

The control group included 20 volunteers (17 male, 3 female, mean age 29±3) enrolled during the same period with similar male/female ratio. Histories, physical examination, ECG, chest radiography and routine chemical analysis showed that the controls had no evidence of coronary heart diseases.

The exclusive criteria were as follows: venous thrombosis, history of severe renal or hepatic diseases, haematological disorders, acute or chronic inflammatory diseases and malignancy.

The study protocol was approved by the ethics committee of Tongji University and informed consent form was obtained.

Gene expression chips

Agilent G4112F Whole Human Genome Oligo Microarrays were purchased from Agilent (USA). A microarray is composed of more than 41,000 genes or transcripts, including targeted 19,596 entrez gene RNAs. Sequence information used in the microarrays is derived from the latest databases of RefSeq, Goldenpath, Ensembl and Unigene. The functions of more than 70% of the genes in the microarray are already known. All patients were subjected to chip analyses. 21,910 probes which detected (with a flag 'P')[5] in all 20 samples of at least one condition were selected for further analysis.

Total RNA isolation

5 ml of peripheral blood samples with PAXgene tube was drawn from patients of AMI and SA, immediately after admission. Leucocytes were obtained through density gradient centrifugation with Ficoll solution and the remaining red blood cells were destroyed by erythrocyte lysis buffer (Qiagen, Hilden, Germany). Total RNA was extracted and purified using PAXgeneTM Blood RNA kit (Cat#762174, QIAGEN, GmBH, Germany), following the manufacturer's instructions. It was further checked for a RIN number to inspect RNA integration by an Agilent Bioanalyzer 2100 (Agilent technologies, Santa Clara, CA, US). The sample was considered qualified when 2100 RIN $\geq$ 7.0 as well as 28S/18S $\geq$ 0.7.

RNA amplification and labeling

Total RNA was amplified and labeled by Low Input Quick Amp Labeling Kit, One-Color (Cat#5190-2305, Agilent technologies, Santa Clara, CA, US), following manufacturer's instructions. Labeled cRNA were purified by RNeasy mini kit (Cat#74106, QIAGEN, GmBH, Germany).

Microarray hybridization

Each slide was hybridized with 1.65μg Cy3-labeled cRNA using Gene Expression Hybridization Kit (Cat#5188-5242, Agilent technologies, Santa Clara, CA, US) in Hybridization Oven (Cat#G2545A, Agilent technologies, Santa Clara, CA, US), following the manufacturer's instructions. After 17 hours of hybridization, slides were washed in staining dishes (Cat#121, Thermo Shandon, Waltham, MA, US) with Gene Expression Wash Buffer Kit(Cat#5188-5327, Agilent technologies, Santa Clara, CA, US) , according to the manufacturer's operation manual.

Chip scan and Data acquisition

Slides were scanned by Agilent Microarray Scanner (Cat#G2565CA, Agilent technologies, Santa Clara, CA, US) with default settings, Dye channel: Green, Scan resolution=3μm,

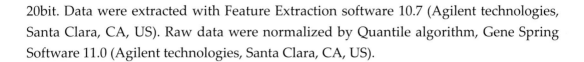

20bit. Data were extracted with Feature Extraction software 10.7 (Agilent technologies, Santa Clara, CA, US). Raw data were normalized by Quantile algorithm, Gene Spring Software 11.0 (Agilent technologies, Santa Clara, CA, US).

RT-PCR

The spots in the microarray were randomly selected and their expressions were confirmed by RT-PCR. Among genes with differential expressions, 3 genes were randomly selected, and these gens and the house keeping genes (GAPDH) were subjected to RT-PCR. The relative expressions were indicated as the expression of the target genes normalized to the expression of GAPDH (2-$\Delta\Delta$Ct). The melting curve and the 2-$\Delta\Delta$Ct-method were used to detect the differences in the expressions among the three groups. The results from RT-PCR were consistent with the microarray analysis.

Data analysis

Firstly, at least one group of genes containing all significant P values was selected from three groups, and a total of 21910 probes were selected [5]. R package "WGCNA" was used to construct the weighted gene co-expression network.[6] First, a matrix of signed Spearman correlations between all probe pairs was computed. Second, this correlation matrix was rising to a power β=16 to calculate an adjacency matrix. The power was determined in WGCNA by making use of the fact that gene expression networks exhibit an approximate scale free topology [7]. Raising the power highlights the strong correlations and mitigates the confounding weak correlations on an exponential scale. We applied the Dynamic Tree Cut algorithm [8] with default parameters to cut the hierarchical tree since co-expression gene modules were defined as branches of the tree. The expression profile of a given module was represented by its first principal component (module eigengene, ME) which can explain the most variation of the module expression levels. Principal Component Analysis (PCA) is commonly used data reduction statistical procedure, which uses an orthogonal transformation to convert observations of correlated underlying variables into a small number of values of linearly uncorrelated variables.[9] Modules with highly correlated module eigengenes (r> 0.85) were merged together to maximize the value of the first principal component and the explained variations. The correlation of sample conditions and MEs were calculated to represent the relevancy of modules and sample conditions. Functions of each module were analyzed via DAVID (Database for Annotation, Visualization and Integrated Discovery).[10]

Results

In the present study, we firstly did the sample clustering of 21910 probes detected in each of the 20 subjects. The clustering of the three groups (Figure 11-1-1) suggested the disease-specific gene expression pattern in AAT. Sample cluster was based on the Spearman correlation of each subject. Dendrograms at the top and left of correlation matrix were hierarchical clustering of all samples while condition cluster was based

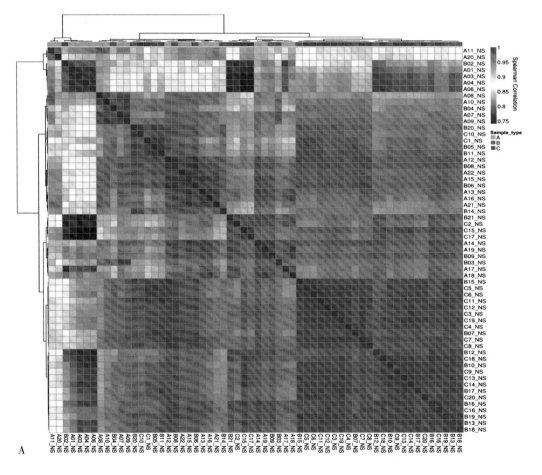

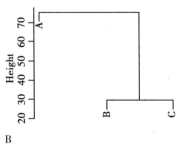

Figure 11-1-1   Sample clustering for three groups, including AMI (A), SAP (B) and 20 healthy volunteers (C). (I) Dendrograms at the top and left of correlation matrix were hierarchical clustering of samples. (II) Condition cluster based on average signal intensity of each probe. The color of each cell symbolized the Spearman correlation of each sample pairs, from high (red) to low (blue). The color band above the correlation matrix is the symbols of sample condition: A(gold), B (red) and C (blue). (Journal of Geriatric Cardiology,2015,12: 287-293)

on average signal intensity of each probe. Then the hierarchical cluster tree showed co-expression modules which were identified using R package "WGCNA" (Figure 11-1-2). Modules corresponded to branches and were labelled by colors as indicated by the first color band underneath the tree. The cluster tree showed the significant differences in co-expression between A and B/C, suggesting the disease-specific gene expression pattern in AAT.

In order to demonstrate the detailed disease-specific gene expressions in AAT, a heatmap of correlations and corresponding p-values between modules and conditions was estimated (Figure 11-1-3). Each module was represented by its module eigengene. Among distinct groups (columns), in A group 4 modules were negatively correlated, while 3 were positively correlated (all P<0.05). Color of each cell indicates the level of

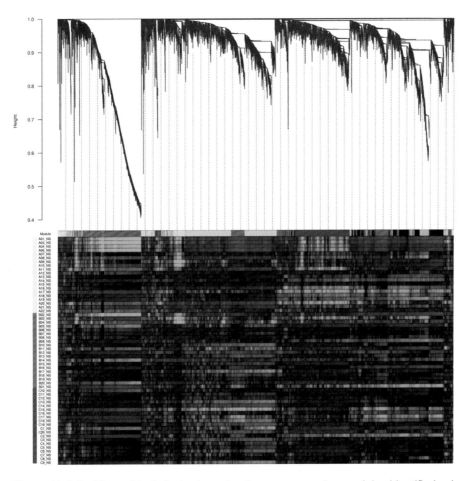

Figure 11-1-2   Hierarchical cluster tree showing co-expression modules identified using WGCNA.Remaining color bands represented the high signal intensity (red) or the low signal intensity (green) probes for each sample. The color band on the left indicated conditions: A (gold), B (red) and C (blue). (Journal of Geriatric Cardiology,2015,12: 287-293)

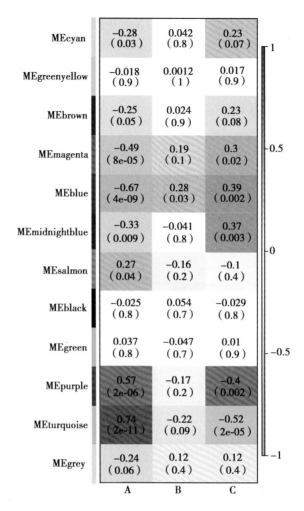

Figure 11-1-3 Heatmap of correlations and corresponding p-values between modules and conditions. Module trait gene represented function of the corresponding module. Figures in boxes represented correlation coefficient between modules and conditions, as well as their P values. Color of boxes: positive correlation (red); negative correlation (green); no correlation (white). Several modules (row) were significant (P<0.05) positive (turquoise) or negative (blue) correlated with different conditions (line). (Journal of Geriatric Cardiology,2015,12: 287-293)

correlation between gene co-expressions with condition specific expression. The blue module was significantly negatively correlated (r=–0.67,P=4e-9), and in the magenta module (r=–0.49, P=8e-5). The turquoise module was highly positively correlated (r=0.74, P =2e-11), and in purple module (r=0.57,P =2e-6).

We chose these four differentially expressed modules to show the functions of genes, as displayed in Figure 11-1-4. The methods of GO terms were used to show the enriched functions. The blue and magenta modules included mitochondrion, negative regulation of cell death, lymphocyte activation, regulation of T cell activation and

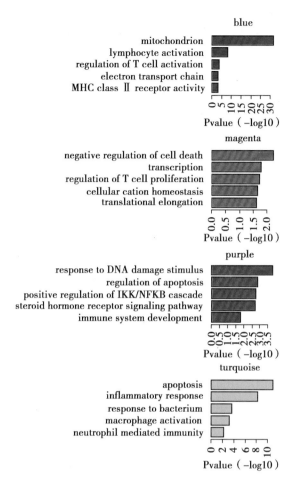

Figure 11-1-4   Enriched function in 4 modules. Bargraph showed the Benjamani-Hochberg adjusted p values (–log10 transferred).

(Journal of Geriatric Cardiology,2015,12: 287-293)

proliferation and so on, while the purple and turquoise modules contained responses to DNA damage stimulus, apoptosis, inflammatory response, response to bacterium, macrophage activation and so on (see Figure 11-1-4).

The sample clustering showed long distance between A and B/C and short distance between B and C, suggesting the disease-specific gene expression pattern in AAT. Hierarchical cluster tree analysis was done to classify all the genes into several co-expression modules, and significant differences were observed in the co-expression modules between A and B/C. Co-expression modules analysis showed that the expressions of some genes were markedly different in A group from that in B group and C group. Genes with significantly down-regulated expression in A group were mainly related to mitochondrion, lymphocyte activation, regulation of T cell activation electron transport chain, MHC class Ⅱ receptor activity, negative regulation of cell death, transcription, regulation of T cell proliferation, cellular cation homeostasis and translational elongation. Genes with significantly up-regulated expressions in A group were mainly associated with response to DNA damage stimulus, regulation of apoptosis, positive regulation of IKK/NFKB cascade, steroid hormone receptor signaling pathway, immune system development, apoptosis, inflammatory response, response to bacterium, macrophage activation and neutrophil mediated immunity.

Biological function analysis of gene expression modules with significant differences showed the injury to cells and tissues, reduced mitochondrial metabolism, compromised ion balance, decreased T cells function, declined activity of CD_4 receptor, increased cell apoptosis, increased inflammation, elevated phagocytosis, elevated neutrophil-mediated immunity and increased post-traumatic repair of cells and tissues in A group.

Coronary arterial thrombosis causes acute myocardial ischemia and hypoxia, injury and necrosis of myocytes, disordered energy metabolism and ion metabolism. Elevated repair of tissues and cells by protein synthesis, increased inflammatory reaction and elevated activity of phagocytes is a reflection of the pathophysiological changes after injury and necrosis of cells and tissues.

In A group, the biological functions of differentially expressed genes were associated to compromised immune function, which was characterized by reduced T cells function, inhibited proliferation of T cells, and reduced activity of MHC class II receptor. CD_3 positive cells refer to total T cells and play a central role in the immunity. CD_3 positive T cells can differentiate into CD_4 T cells and CD_8 T cells. CD_4 T cells may accept signals after antigen presenting and secret different cytokines to combat with different pathogens and assist B cell activity. CD_8 T cells may directly kill the cells infected by virus/bacterium, allogeneic cells and cancer cells [11,12]. NK cells are a participant of innate immunity, belong to T cells differentiated from primitive macrophages and have similar killing function to CD_8 T cells [13].

In A group, the T cells function was significantly compromised, suggesting the collapse of immune defense. What is the consequence of the collapse of immune defense? Under this condition, the human body fails to effectively and timely clear foreign pathogenic microorganisms and endogenous cancer cells. In the present study, cancers were excluded from these subjects. Thus, we speculated that the pathogenesis of AAT was related to the inflammatory reaction after arterial intima infection caused by potential pathogenic microorganisms in human body.

The pathogenesis of AAT is closely related to significantly compromised functions of T cells, an important participant of immunity in human body. Our findings provide new evidence on the pathogenesis of AAT.

(published:Journal of Geriatric Cardiology (2015) 12: 287-293)

References

1. Kashyap VS, Reil TD, Moore WS, Hoang TX, Gelabert HA, Byrns RE, Ignarro LJ, Freischlag JA. Acute arterial thrombosis causes endothelial dysfunction: a new paradigm for thrombolytic therapy.J Vasc Surg. 2001;34(2):323-9.

2. Rautou PE, Vion AC, Amabile N, Chironi G, Simon A, Tedgui A, Boulanger CM. Microparticles, vascular function, and atherothrombosis. Circ Res.2011 Aug 19;109(5):593-606.

3. Siddiqui TI, Kumar K S A, Dikshit DK.Platelets and atherothrombosis: causes, targets and treatments for thrombosis.Curr Med Chem.2013;20(22):2779-97.

4. Thygesen K, Alpert JS, Jaffe AS, Simoons ML, Chaitman BR, White HD, et al.Third universal definition of myocardial infarction.J Am Coll Cardiol. 2012 ;60(16):1581-98.

5. Pepper SD, Saunders EK, Edwards LE, Wilson CL, Miller CJ: The utility of MAS5 expression summary and detection call algorithms. BMC bioinformatics ,2007;8:273.

6. Langfelder P, Horvath S: WGCNA: an R package for weighted correlation network analysis. BMC bioinformatics .2008;9:559.

7. Albert R, Jeong H, Barabasi AL. Error and attack tolerance of complex networks.Nature .2000; 406:378-382.

8. Langfelder P, Horvath S: Fast R Functions for Robust Correlations and Hierarchical Clustering. Journal of statistical software .2012;46(11).

9. Jolliffe, Ian. Principal component analysis. John Wiley & Sons, Ltd, 2002.

10. Huang da W, Sherman BT, Lempicki RA: Systematic and integrative analysis of large gene lists using DAVID bioinformatics resources. Nature protocols. 2009;4(1):44-57.

11. McKinstry KK, Strutt TM, Swain SL.Regulation of CD_4 T-cell contraction during pathogen challenge.Immunol Rev. 2010;236:110-24.

12. Gadhamsetty S, Marée AF, Beltman JB, de Boer RJ.A general functionLal response of cytotoxic T lymphocyte-mediated killing of target cells. Biophys J. 2014 ;106(8):1780-91.

13. Sun JC, Lanier LL.NK cell development, homeostasis and function: parallels with CD_8 T cells. Nat Rev Immunol. 2011;11(10):645-57.

Chapter 12

Human genomics in patients with acute myocardial infarction

1. Expression characteristics of neutrophil and mononuclear-phagocyte related genes in patients with AMI and SAP

Inflammatory reaction goes through the entire occurrence, development and evolution of coronary atherosclerosis and affects the stability and natural process of atherosclerotic plaque to some extent [1]. As the most important inflammatory cells, phagocytes including neutrophils and monocytes directly participate in atherosclerosis and the occurrence and development of acute coronary events with a variety of inflammatory factors.[2]

It has been shown that absolute neutrophil count among patients with acute myocardial infarction (AMI) was obviously higher than that among the stable angina pectoris (SAP) and control group. Moreover, there exist striking expressions of inflammatory factors and infiltration of neutrophils and macrophages in unstable plaques [3,4]. Activated neutrophils can prompt the progress of atheromatous plaque and increase its instability through chemotaxis, degranulation and oxidative stress and so on [5]. Monocyte adhesion to vascular endothelial cells initiates atherosclerosis, and activates monocytes into macrophages, further accelerating the formation of foam cells and plaques [6]. Many PRRs, opsonic receptors and cytokine receptors are expressed on the surface of neutrophils and macrophages, which are closely related to the adhesive, chemotactic and phagocytic functions of neutrophils and monocytes-macrophages and can increase plaque instability by many immunoinflammatory factors.

Whole Human Genome Oligo Microarrays were applied to detect expression differences of neutrophil and monocyte-macrophage function related genes in AMI, SAP and control groups.

Patient information

This prospective study included three groups of patients with a total of 60 subjects, including 20 patients with AMI, 20 with SA, and 20 healthy volunteers. The baseline demographic data are displayed in Table 12-1-1. The AMI patients were admitted <12 hours from the onset of symptoms to our coronary care unit between January and June 2013, including 18 males and 2 females, with an average age of 58±12 years. All AMI subjects were diagnosed on the basis of the following criteria: Detection of a rise of cardiac biomarker values [preferably cardiac troponin (cTn)] with at least one value above the 99th percentile upper reference limit (URL) and with at least one of the following: 1) Symptoms of ischemia; 2) New or presumed new significant ST-segment-T wave (ST-T) changes or new left bundle branch block (LBBB); 3) Development of pathological Q waves in the ECG; 4) Imaging evidence of new loss of viable myocardium or new regional wall motion abnormality; and 5) Identification of an intracoronary thrombus by angiography.

In the SAP group, 20 patients (18 males, 2 females, mean age 64±10 years) with exclusively effort-related angina were studied, with a positive exercise stress test and at least one coronary stenosis detected at angiography (>70% reduction of lumen diameter). There were no significant differences between AMI and SAP patients in age, gender, smoking, BMI, systolic blood pressure, diastolic blood pressure, LDL-C, triglycerides, HDL-C and fasting plasma glucose (FPG) (see Table1 2-1-1).

Table 12-1-1   Baseline demographic data in three groups (mean±s. d.)

	AMI(a)(N=20)	SA (b)(N=20)	Con(c)(N=20)	P(all)	P(a v b)
Age(years)	57.8±11.9	63.6±9.9	28.8±3.3	0.000	0.251
Sex(M/F)	18/2	18/2	17/3	0.853	1.0
BMI(kg/m^2)	23.6±2.6	22.8±2.7	21.3±1.8	0.102	0.56
Smoke(NO./d)	13.6±12.2	9.8±10.3	0	0.00	0.648
Syst(mmHg)	128.6±15.3	123.0±12.1	120.8±7.2	0.115	0.501
Diast(mmHg)	67.0±8.0	73.0±8.0	71.6±3.2	0.017	0.064
LDL-C(mmol/L)	2.5±1.0	2.1±0.8	2.9±0.5	0.327	0.548
Triglycerides(mmol/L)	1.6±1.1	1.5±1.4	1.2±0.4	0.73	0.762
HDL-C(mmol/L)	0.8±0.7	0.9±0.2	1.3±0.2	0.000	0.803
FPG(mmol/L)	5.4±0.9	5.0±0.8	4.9±0.5	0.61	0.082
Scr(μmol/L)	87.2±19.6	76.9±14.8	72.2±6.4	0.327	0.138

The control group included 20 volunteers (17 males and 3 females, mean age 29±3 years) enrolled during the same period with similar male/female ratio. Histories, physical examination, ECG, chest radiography and routine chemical analysis showed the controls had no evidence of coronary heart diseases.

The exclusive criteria for the three groups were as follows: venous thrombosis, history of severe renal or hepatic diseases, haematological disorders, acute or chronic inflammatory diseases and malignancy.

The study protocol was approved by the local ethics committee of Tongji University and informed consent form was also obtained.

Gene expression clip

Agilent G4112F Whole Human Genome Oligo Microarrays were purchased from Agilent (USA). A microarray is composed of more than 41000 genes or transcripts, including targeted 19,596 entrez gene RNAs. Sequence information used in the microarrays was derived from the latest databases of RefSeq, Goldenpath, Ensembl and Unigene. The functions of more than 70% of the genes in the microarray are already known. All patients were subjected to clip analysis.

Total RNA isolation

5 ml of peripheral blood samples with PAXgene tube were drawn from patients of AMI and SA, immediately after being admitted to the hospital, and did the same to the controls. Leucocytes were obtained through density gradient centrifugation with Ficoll solution and the remaining red blood cells were destroyed by erythrocyte lysis buffer (Qiagen, Hilden, Germany). Total RNA was extracted and purified using PAXgene^{TM} Blood RNA kit (Cat#762174, QIAGEN, GmBH, Germany) following the manufacturer's instructions and checked for a RIN number to inspect RNA integration by an Agilent Bioanalyzer 2100 (Agilent technologies, Santa Clara, CA, US). The sample was considered qualified when 2100 RIN$\geqslant$7.0 as well as 28S/18S$\geqslant$0.7.

RNA amplification and labeling

Total RNA was amplified and labeled by Low Input Quick Amp Labeling Kit, One-Color (Cat#5190-2305, Agilent technologies, Santa Clara, CA, US), following the manufacturer's instructions. Labeled cRNA were purified by RNeasy mini kit (Cat#74106, QIAGEN, GmBH, Germany).

Microarray hybridization

Each Slide was hybridized with 1.65μg Cy3-labeled cRNA using Gene Expression Hybridization Kit (Cat#5188-5242, Agilent technologies, Santa Clara, CA, US) in Hybridization Oven (Cat#G2545A, Agilent technologies, Santa Clara, CA, US), followed the manufacturer's instructions. After 17 hours hybridization, slides were washed in staining dishes (Cat#121, Thermo Shandon, Waltham, MA, US) with Gene Expression Wash Buffer Kit(Cat#5188-5327, Agilent technologies, Santa Clara, CA, US),according to the manufacturer's operation manual.

Chip scan and Data acquisition

Slides were scanned by Agilent Microarray Scanner (Cat#G2565CA, Agilent technologies, Santa Clara, CA, US) with default settings, Dye channel: Green, Scan resolution=3μm, 20bit. Data were extracted with Feature Extraction software 10.7 (Agilent technologies, Santa Clara, CA, US). Raw data were normalized by Quantile algorithm, Gene Spring Software 11.0 (Agilent technologies, Santa Clara, CA, US).

RT-PCR

The spots in the microarray were randomly selected and their expressions were confirmed by RT-PCR. Among genes with differential expressions, 3 genes were randomly selected, and these gens and the house keeping genes (GAPDH) were subjected to RT-PCR. The relative expressions were indicated as the expression of the target genes normalized to the expression of GAPDH ($2\text{-}\Delta\Delta Ct$). The melting curve and the $2\text{-}\Delta\Delta Ct$-method were used to compare the differences in the expressions among three groups. The results from RT-PCR were consistent with the microarray analysis.

Statistical analysis

Values were expressed as mean±S.E.M. Groups differences were examined by one-way analysis of variance (ANOVA).Pair-wise group comparisons after ANOVA were performed using Tukey's multiple comparison technique. Data were analyzed using SPSS 19.0, and p-values <0.05 were considered statistically significant.

Results

CSFs and their receptors related mRNAs expression

Total mRNAs of seven CSFs and their receptors were detected. Compared with the controls: (1) mRNAs of all CSFs and their receptors were up-regulated in the AMI group, and the expression of GM-CSFRA and G-CSFR mRNAs was significantly up-regulated (P<0.01); and (2) 6 of all 7 mRNAs were up-regulated in the SAP group, and GM-CSFRA mRNA expression was significantly up-regulated (P<0.05). M-CSFR mRNA was down-regulated without significant difference. Compared with the SAP group, mRNAs of CSFs and their receptors were up-regulated in the AMI group, and the expression of GM-CSFRA and G-CSFR was significantly up-regulated (P<0.01) (Figure 12-1-1).

Expression of main chemokines and their receptors

Total mRNAs of 6 chemokines and their receptors were detected. Compared with the controls: (1) 4 mRNAs were significantly up-regulated in the AMI group (CCR2, CCL2/MCP-1 and CXCR2 mRNAs expression P<0.01; IL8 mRNA expression P<0.05), and 2 CCL3/MIP-1 mRNAs expression was down-regulated without significant difference. (2) mRNAs of all chemokines and their receptors in the SAP group showed an upward

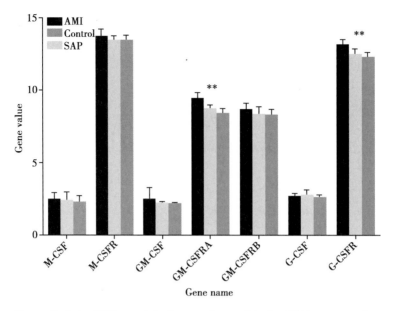

Figure12-1-1 CSFs and their receptors related mRNAs expression
(*P<0.05, **P<0.01) (Journal of Geriatric Cardiology,2015,12: 279-286)

trend, and CCR2 mRNA was significantly up-regulated(P<0.01). Compared with the SAP group, the expression of CCR2, CCL2/MCP-1 and CXCR2 was significantly up-regulated (P<0.01) (Figure 12-1-2).

Opsonic receptors related mRNAs expression

Total mRNAs of 6 opsonic receptors related were detected. Compared with the controls: (1) all opsonic receptors (IgG FcR and C3bR/C4bR) were significantly up-regulated (P<0.01) in the AMI group. (2) All mRNAs in the SAP group were also up-

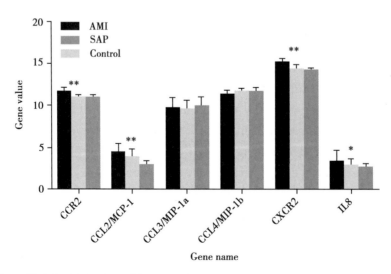

Figure12-1-2 Main chemokines and their receptors related mRNAs expression
(*P<0.05, **P<0.01) (Journal of Geriatric Cardiology,2015,12: 279-286)

regulated (FCGR2B mRNA expression P<0.05). Compared with the controls, mRNAs of all opsonic receptors were significantly up-regulated (FCGR2A, FCGR2B, FCGR3A, FCGR3B and CR1 mRNAs expression P<0.01) in the AMI group (Figure 12-1-3).

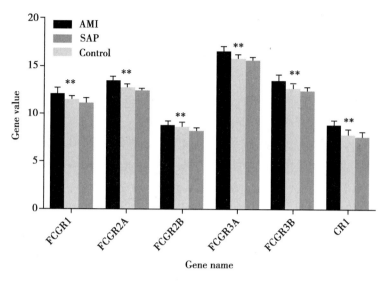

Figure 12-1-3   Opsonic receptors related mRNAs expression (*P<0.05, **P<0.01) (Journal of Geriatric Cardiology,2015,12: 279-286)

PRR related mRNAs expression

Total mRNAs of 12 PRR were detected. Compared with the controls: (1) 11 PRR were up-regulated in the AMI group, and 9 mRNAs (MSR,TLR1,2,4-6,8-10) of them were significantly up-regulated (P<0.01); (2) 10 PRR related mRNAs were up-regulated in the SAP group (TLR2, 5 mRNAs expression P<0.01, TLR6 mRNA expression P<0.05), MRC and TLR9 mRNA expression was down-regulated without significant difference. Compared with the SAP group, 11 mRNAs expression was significantly up-regulated (TLR1, 2, 4-6, 8-10 mRNA expression P<0.01, MRC mRNA expression P<0.05)(Figure 12-1-4).

Inflammatory reaction plays an important role in different stages of coronary atherosclerosis, including the formation, stability, progress, and rupture of plaques and acute thrombosis [1]. As the most important inflammatory cells, neutrophil and mononuclear-macrophages and inflammatory factors work together to promote atherosclerosis and the occurrence and development of acute coronary events [2]. It has been shown that the adhesive, chemotactic and phagocytic functions of neutrophils and mononuclear-macrophages are closely related to many cytokines and receptors, which are expressed on their own surface [7,8].

CSFs and their receptors related mRNAs expression

Colony-stimulating factor (G-CSF) is a multifunctional cytokine, which can stimulate

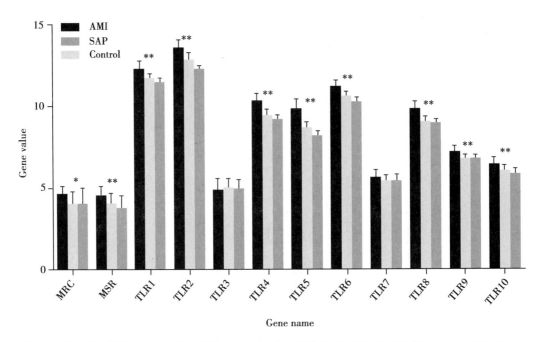

Figure 12-1-4   PRRs related mRNAs expression (*P<0.05, **P<0.01) (Journal of Geriatric Cardiology,2015,12: 279-286)

the proliferation and differentiation of pluripotent hematopoietic stem cells and hemopoietic progenitor cells in different development stages. It includes granulocyte-macrophage colony stimulating factor (GM-CSF), macrophage colony stimulating factor (M-CSF), granulocyte colony stimulating factor (G-CSF), erythropoietin (EPO), thrombopoietin (TPO) and so on. M-CSF can induce hematopoietic progenitor cells to differentiate into mononuclear cells and macrophages, and increase the expression of scavenger receptor on the macrophage surface to promote the AS process [9]. GM-CSF mainly promotes the proliferation and differentiation of granulocytes and macrophages, enhances the adhesive, chemotactic and phagocytic functions of neutrophils and mononuclear cells, strengthen the adhesion and infiltration of monocyte-macrophages to endothelial cells, and then promote the AS inflammatory reaction [10]. G-CSF can adjust specifically the proliferation and differentiation of granulocyte, strengthen the function of mature granulocytes, increase the number of neutrophils, and promote inflammation [11]. The results of this study showed that: almost all colony-stimulating factors (CSF) and their receptors were up-regulated in the AMI and SAP groups compared with the control group, and the expression of GM-CSFR and G-CSFR in the AMI group was significantly up-regulated than in the SAP and control groups (P<0.01), suggesting that CSF is expressed obviously in coronary AS inflammatory reaction, and the expression of CSF shows a stepped upward trend as the disease progresses.

mRNAs expression of main chemokines and their receptors

Chemokines and their receptors play important roles in activation and migration of inflammatory cells and are contributing factors in the progression of AS. Studies have shown that the occurrence and development of coronary atherosclerotic heart disease (CHD) are closely related to main chemokines such as monocyte chemotactic protein-1(MCP-1), macrophage inflammatory protein-1(MIP-1) and IL-8 [11-14]. These chemokines can enhance the chemotaxis and activation of neutrophils and monocytes, induce macrophages to release inflammatory mediators, promote endothelial cell activation and the expression of adhesion molecules, promote monocyte adhesion and infiltration on vascular endothelial cells and then transform into macrophages to swallow lipid, finally lead to foam cell and plaque formation. In this study, we found that the expression of mRNAs related to monocyte chemoattractant protein-1(MCP-1), CCR2 (MCP-1 receptor) and CXCR2 (IL-8 receptor) was significantly up-regulated in the AMI group compared with the SAP and control groups (P<0.01), and IL-8 mRNA expression in the AMI group was clearly higher (P<0.05) than the controls.

The results indicate that the chemokines MCP-1 and IL-8 are closely related to the occurrence and development of AS and acute ischemic events; moreover, the expression of MCP-1 and IL-8 shows a stepped upward trend as the disease progresses.

Opsonic receptors and PRR related mRNAs expression

Epidemiological and clinicopathologic studies have suggested that infectious agents such as bacteria, viruses and chlamydia are associated with the occurrence and development of AS and coronary heart disease.[15,16]　Infectious agents may initiate and maintain inflammatory response through innate immune and play roles in the formation and development of atherosclerosis. Studies have suggested that in innate immune, opsonic receptors (IgG FcR and C3bR/C4bR) and pattern recognition receptors (MR, MSR, TLR) in the surface of neutrophils and mononuclear-macrophages play important roles in the progression of AS and CAD through mediating Inflammation [17-19].

The results of this study showed that: (1) all the mRNAs related to opsonic receptors (IgG FcR and C3bR/C4bR) expression were significantly up-regulated (P<0.01) in the AMI group compared with SAP and control groups, and the SAP group showed an upward trend compared with the controls. (2) Most PRR related mRNAs expression was up-regulated in AMI group compared with SAP and control groups. Most TLR mRNAs expression was significantly up-regulated compared to the SAP and control groups except TLR3 and TLR7(P<0.01); TLR2, 5, 6 mRNAs were significantly up-regulated (P<0.05) in SAP group compared with the control group.

MSR mRNA was significantly up-regulated (P<0.01) in AMI group compared with the control group. The results indicated that in the progression of CAD, especially AMI, (1) opsonic receptors mRNAs expression is significantly up-regulated in neutrophils and mononuclear-macrophages, which can enhance the phagocytosis of phagocytes and promote inflammatory response obviously; (2) PRR mRNAs expression in mononuclear-macrophages is significantly up-regulated. MSR can strengthen the adhesion and aggregation of monocytes to vascular endothelial cells, and then promote the inflammation in atherosclerosis area. Besides, MSR plays an important role in macrophage foam cell formation by promoting macrophage to swallow oxidized low density lipoprotein (ox LDL) [20]. TLRs activate signal transduction pathways such as the pathways of NF-κβ and mitogen-activated protein kinase (MAPK) after binding related ligands, and initiate mRNA transcription of inflammatory cytokines and promote inflammation through inducing mononuclear cells gathered to atherosclerosis [17].

In the process of coronary atherosclerosis and AMI, functionally related genes mRNAs expression in neutrophils and mononuclear-macrophages was up-regulated and significantly up-regulated, including CSF and their receptors, chemokines and their receptors, opsonic receptors, PRR. This result suggested that the enhancement of adhesive, chemotactic and phagocytic functions in neutrophils and mononuclear-macrophages goes through the entire occurrence, development of CAD; moreover, this function enhancement will become more remarkable with the deterioration of coronary atherosclerosis disease.

(published: Journal of Geriatric Cardiology (2015) 12: 279-286)

References

1. Libby P: Inflammation in atherosclerosis. Arteriosclerosis, thrombosis, and vascular biology 2012, 32(9):2045-2051.

2. Legein B, Temmerman L, Biessen EA, Lutgens E: Inflammation and immune system interactions in atherosclerosis. Cellular and molecular life sciences: CMLS 2013, 70(20):3847-3869.

3. Dogan I, Karaman K, Sonmez B, Celik S, Turker O: Relationship between serum neutrophil count and infarct size in patients with acute myocardial infarction. Nuclear medicine communications 2009, 30(10):797-801.

4. Tavora FR, Ripple M, Li L, Burke AP: Monocytes and neutrophils expressing myeloperoxidase occur in fibrous caps and thrombi in unstable coronary plaques. BMC cardiovascular disorders 2009, 9:27.

5. Drechsler M, Doring Y, Megens RT, Soehnlein O: Neutrophilic granulocytes-promiscuous accelerators of atherosclerosis. Thrombosis and haemostasis 2011, 106(5):839-848.

6. Andres V, Pello OM, Silvestre-Roig C: Macrophage proliferation and apoptosis in atherosclerosis. Current opinion in lipidology 2012, 23(5):429-438.

7. Xing L, Remick DG: Relative cytokine and cytokine inhibitor production by mononuclear cells and neutrophils. Shock (Augusta, Ga) 2003, 20(1):10-16.

8. Thomas CJ, Schroder K: Pattern recognition receptor function in neutrophils. Trends in immunology 2013, 34(7):317-328.

9. Di Gregoli K, Johnson JL: Role of colony-stimulating factors in atherosclerosis. Current opinion in lipidology 2012,

23(5):412-421.

10. Huang HQ, Wang XX: [Advances in new clinical application of recombinant human granulocyte-macrophage colony-stimulating factor]. Zhonghua xue ye xue za zhi = Zhonghua xueyexue zazhi 2012, 33(5):429-431.

11. Molineux G: Granulocyte colony-stimulating factors. Cancer treatment and research 2011, 157:33-53.

12. Sekalska B: [Aortic expression of monocyte chemotactic protein-1 (MCP-1) gene in rabbits with experimental atherosclerosis]. Annales Academiae Medicae Stetinensis 2003, 49:79-90.

13. istnes M: Macrophage inflammatory protein-1beta: a novel prognostic biomarker in atherosclerosis? Cardiology 2012, 121(3):149-151.

14. Papadopoulou C, Corrigall V, Taylor PR, Poston RN: The role of the chemokines MCP-1, GRO-alpha, IL-8 and their receptors in the adhesion of monocytic cells to human atherosclerotic plaques. Cytokine 2008, 43(2):181-186.

15. Kurano M, Tsukamoto K: [Etiology of atherosclerosis-special reference to bacterial infection and viral infection]. Nihon rinsho Japanese journal of clinical medicine 2011, 69(1):25-29.

16. Syrovatka P, Kraml P: [Infection and atherosclerosis]. Vnitrni lekarstvi 2007, 53(3):286-291.

17. Krejsek J, Kunes P, Andrys C, Holicka M, Novosad J, Kudlova M, Kolackova M: [Innate immunity, receptors for exogenous and endogenous danger patterns in immunopathogenesis of atherosclerosis--part II: TLR receptors, significance of genetic polymorphism of danger signals receptors]. Casopis lekaru ceskych 2005, 144(12):790-794.

18. Oude Nijhuis MM, van Keulen JK, Pasterkamp G, Quax PH, de Kleijn DP: Activation of the innate immune system in atherosclerotic disease. Current pharmaceutical design 2007, 13(10):983-994.

19. Durst R, Neumark Y, Meiner V, Friedlander Y, Sharon N, Polak A, Beeri R, Danenberg H, Erez G, Spitzen S et al: Increased risk for atherosclerosis of various macrophage scavenger receptor 1 alleles. Genetic testing and molecular biomarkers 2009, 13(5):583-587.

20. Kzhyshkowska J, Neyen C, Gordon S: Role of macrophage scavenger receptors in atherosclerosis. Immunobiology 2012, 217(5):492-502.

2. Expression characteristics of natural killer cell related genes mRNA in patients with AMI and SAP

Natural killer (NK) cell is a key cellular component of innate immune response characterized by strong cytolytic activity against susceptible target cells and the ability to release several cytokines. NK cells provide the first-line defense against infecting microbes, tumors and autoimmune diseases [1]. Although NK cells do not express classical antigen receptors of the immunoglobulin-gene family, such as the antibodies produced by B cells or the T cell receptors expressed by T cells, they use an array of innate receptors to sense their environment and respond to alterations caused by infections, cellular stress, and transformation. No single activation receptor dominates; instead, synergistic signals from combinations of inhibitory and activating receptors are integrated to activate natural cytotoxicity and cytokine production [2].

Important roles of NK cell function in atherosclerosis [3] are reflected by the significant reduction of circulating NK cell numbers with a concomitant loss in NK cell function in patients with non-STEMI, unstable or stable coronary artery diseases [4-6]. Jonasson suggested that the impaired NK cell function in patients with coronary atherosclerosis diseases (CAD) might be a mainly quantitative defect [4]. Li et al presented that the rate of spontaneous NK cell apoptosis was increased in CAD patients [6], and Backteman et al described that the sustained reduction of NK cells was associated with low-grade inflammation [5]. However, it has not yet been possible to fully explain the mechanisms controlling the suppression of NK cells in CAD, especially, very few studies were performed towards the NK receptors in CAD patients. Therefore, in the present study, human microarray analysis was used to systematically examine the mRNA expressions of NK cell receptors in PBMCs isolated from AMI, SAP patients and controls. We designed this *in vitro* study to investigate the gene expression differences of inhibitory and activating NK cell receptors in patients with AMI and SA.

Results

Gene expressions of inhibitory NK cell receptors

The results showed mRNA expressions of inhibitory NK cell receptors including killer cell immunoglobulin-like receptors (KIRs) and killer lectin-like receptors (KLRs). The KIRs consist of KIR2DL2, KIR2DL5A, KIR3DL1, KIR3DL2, and KIR3DL3, and the KLRs comprise CD94/NKG2A, KLRG1and KLRB1, so nine mRNA expressions of NK cell inhibitory receptors in PBMCs from three groups were detected (Figure 12-2-1). In

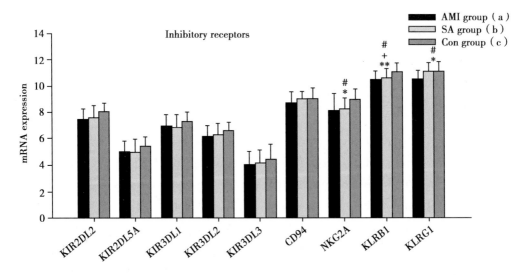

Figure 12-2-1   mRNA expressions of inhibitory NK cell receptors in PBMCs from three groups. Three groups *P<0.05, **P<0.01. (International Journal of Clinical and Experimental Pathology,2015,8(11): 14667-14675)

PBMCs from the three groups, expressions of the genes encoding NKG2A, KLRB1, and KLRG1 were significantly different (P<0.05). In AMI group, all the nine gene expressions were lower and the NKG2A, KLRB1, and KLRG1 mRNA expressions were significantly lower than the controls (P<0.05). Between the SAP and control groups, there was no significant difference in mRNA expressions though seven gene expressions had a downward trend. The mRNA expression of KLRB1 in AMI patients was significantly down-regulated in comparison with the SAP patients (P<0.05).

Gene expressions of activating NK cell receptors

Eleven mRNA expressions of activating NK cell receptors in PBMCs from the three groups were examined (Figure 12-2-2), which included natural cytotoxicity receptors (NCRs), KIRs (NKG2D), the SLAM-related receptors (SRR) and other NK cell activating receptors containing DNAX accessory molecule-1 (DNAM-1), CD2, CD7, and CD96 (Tactile). The NCRs comprise NKp30, NKp44 and NKp46. 2B4 (CD244), NTB-A (CD352), and CRACC (CD319) are members of the recently defined family of SRR. In PBMCs from three groups, expressions of the genes encoding NKp30, NTB-A, CRACC, CD2, CD7, and CD96 were significantly different (P<0.01). In AMI group all the eleven gene expressions of activating receptors were lowest among three groups, and NKp30, NTB-A, CRACC, CD2, CD7, and CD96 mRNAs in AMI patients were significantly down-regulated compared with controls and SAP patients respectively(P<0.05). Between the SA and control group seven gene expressions were lower in SAP patients, but without significant difference.

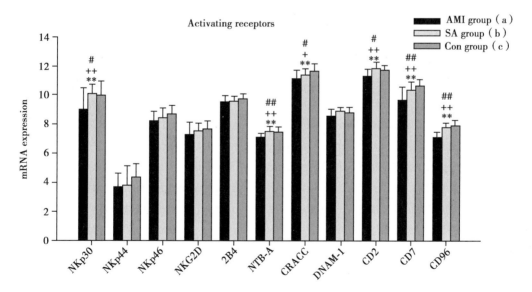

Figure 12-2-2　mRNA expression of activating NK cell receptors in PBMCs from three groups. Three groups *P<0.05, **P<0.01; a vs. c #P<0.05, ##P<0.01. b vs. c &P<0.05, &&P<0.01. a vs. b +P<0.05, ++P<0.01. (International Journal of Clinical and Experimental Pathology,2015,8(11): 14667-14675)

The NK cells express an array of inhibitory and activating receptors, and the inhibitory receptors recognize specific molecules that are expressed on normal cells as a means of protecting them from lysis by NK cells. Classically, inhibitory receptors, for example the KIRs and NKG2A receptors, recognize major histocompatibility complex class I (MHC-I) molecules [7]. Considerable evidences confirm that the signal transmitted by NK inhibitory receptors is dominant together with the activating receptors for the normal cells protection [2]. In our present study, all the seven gene expressions of MHC-I specific-molecule receptors in AMI patients were lower and the NKG2A mRNA expression was significantly lower than the controls, which suggested the declined ability of NK cells in the recognition of MHC-I molecules and the decreased protection of normal cells in AMI patients. Recent works have revealed that there is another system of NK-cell inhibition, which is independent of MHC-I molecules. MHC class I-independent inhibitory receptors such as KLRG1 and KLRB1 play crucial roles in inducing peripheral tolerance, and these newly discovered NK-cell inhibitory receptors have broadened the definition of self as seen by NK cells [8,9]. The mechanism of signals from these receptors is not fully clear, however, clinical studies and animal experiments have shown that these receptors may be related to the prevention of autoimmune diseases [10,11]. During our study, significant down-regulation of KLRG1 and KLRB1 mRNA expressions in AMI group showed the deceased ability to prevent autoimmune disease in AMI patients. As to SAP patients, the gene expressions of inhibitory NK receptors had no significant difference compared with the controls indicating that no initiation of any inhibitory NK receptors is activated in SAP group.

The activating receptors are widely expressed on the surface of NK cells. NCRs including NKp30, NKp44 and NKp46, are one of the most important activating receptors which mediate the NK-cell cytotoxicity. NCRs have been shown to recognize a broad spectrum of ligands ranging from viral-, parasite-and bacterial-derived ligands to cellular ligands and play a central role in eliminating infected or transformed cells, especially malignant cells [12-14]. Another central activating NK cell receptor is NKG2D, which can bind to many ligands that are induced on cells under stress due to infection, transformation, or DNA damage. Therefore, NKG2D has an important role in targeting NK cell responses toward abnormal cells and finally the lysis [15,16]. Like NKG2D ligands, DNAM-1 ligands are frequently expressed on stressed cells, and DNAM-1 receptor participates in a cytotoxic immune response when binding to their ligands [17-19]. The 2B4, NTB-A and CRACC receptors belong to the family of SRR and transmit activating signals through the SLAM-associated protein (SAP) [20]. Many other receptors, including CD2, CD7 and CD96, can contribute to NK cell activation, but much work remains to be done in determining how and when the various NK cell receptors deliver signals for activation [2,21]. Among the activating receptors, the most dominant NCRs and NKG2D receptors, however, do not activate the NK cells by their own. Activation of NK cells by any of the tested receptors requires complementation with another activating receptor, such as 2B4, NTB-A, CRACC or DNMA-1 to obtain synergistic activation signals, and then releases the perforin and granzyme, leading to the direct target cells lysis [22]. Meanwhile the requirement for combination may serve as a safeguard to prevent unrestrained activation of NK cells [23]. In our study, all the eleven gene expressions of activating receptors in AMI patients were lowest among three groups, and NKp30, NTB-A, CRACC, CD2, CD7 and CD96 mRNAs were significantly decreased in comparison with SAP patients and controls respectively. The results showed that the transduction of activating signal was inhibited in patients with AMI and, as a result, the NK cell immune activity for the targeted cells was decreased. Same as the inhibitory receptors, there was no statistical difference of mRNA expression between the SAP patients and controls about activating receptors, all indicating that the NK receptors in SAP patients were almost in an inactive state.

In the present study, several inhibitory NK cell receptors were significantly lower than the controls and SAP patients, suggesting the decreased ability of normal cells protection in AMI patients. Meanwhile, the significant down-regulated activating NK receptors in AMI group reflect the decline of the immune activity of NK cells. The results of our study demonstrated that the pathogenesis of AMI may be associated with NK cell deficient immune activity or the progress of AMI restrained the NK cell immune activity, however, either side showed the close relationship between AMI and NK cells. There was no statistical distinction of gene expressions in the inhibitory and activating receptors between the SAP patients and controls, showing the apparent differences in NK receptors expressions of AMI and SAP groups. Although previous studies had confirmed the reduced proportions of NK cells in peripheral blood of CAD [5-7], and in line with this, the decreasing NK cell levels were also found in our study from both AMI and SAP patients (data not shown), we can distinguish the differences of NK cell deficit between the numbers and receptor activity in AMI and SAP patients, and the NK cell receptor activity was more decreased in AMI patients.

(published: Int J Clin Exp Pathol 2015;8(11):14667-14675)

References

1. Martin-Fontecha A and Carbone E. The social life of NK cells. Arch Immunol Ther Exp (Warsz) 2001; 49 Suppl 1: S33-9.

2. Long EO, Kim HS, Liu D, Peterson ME and Rajagopalan S. Controlling natural killer cell responses: integration of signals for activation and inhibition. Annu Rev Immunol 2013; 31: 227-58.

3. Whitman SC, Rateri DL, Szilvassy SJ, Yokoyama W and Daugherty A. Depletion of natural killer cell function decreases atherosclerosis in low-density lipoprotein receptor null mice. Arterioscler Thromb Vasc Biol 2004; 24:

1049-54.

4. Jonasson L, Backteman K and Ernerudh J. Loss of natural killer cell activity in patients with coronary artery disease. Atherosclerosis 2005; 183: 316-21.

5. Backteman K, Ernerudh J and Jonasson L. Natural killer (NK) cell deficit in coronary artery disease: no aberrations in phenotype but sustained reduction of NK cells is associated with low-grade inflammation. Clin Exp Immunol 2014; 175: 104-12.

6. Li W, Lidebjer C, Yuan XM, Szymanowski A, Backteman K, Ernerudh J, Leanderson P, Nilsson L, Swahn E and Jonasson L. NK cell apoptosis in coronary artery disease: relation to oxidative stress. Atherosclerosis 2008; 199: 65-72.

7. Moretta L, Bottino C, Pende D, Vitale M, Mingari MC and Moretta A. Different checkpoints in human NK-cell activation. Trends Immunol 2004; 25: 670-6.

8. Kumar V and McNerney ME. A new self: MHC-class-I-independent natural-killer-cell self-tolerance. Nat Rev Immunol 2005; 5: 363-74.

9. Lebbink RJ and Meyaard L. Non-MHC ligands for inhibitory immune receptors: novel insights and implications for immune regulation. Mol Immunol 2007; 44: 2153-64.

10. Ito M, Maruyama T, Saito N, Koganei S, Yamamoto K and Matsumoto N. Killer cell lectin-like receptor G1 binds three members of the classical cadherin family to inhibit NK cell cytotoxicity. J Exp Med 2006; 203: 289-95.

11. Li Y, Hofmann M, Wang Q, Teng L, Chlewicki LK, Pircher H and Mariuzza RA. Structure of natural killer cell receptor KLRG1 bound to E-cadherin reveals basis for MHC-independent missing self recognition. Immunity 2009; 31: 35-46.

12. Kruse PH, Matta J, Ugolini S and Vivier E. Natural cytotoxicity receptors and their ligands. Immunol Cell Biol 2013;

13. Koch J, Steinle A, Watzl C and Mandelboim O. Activating natural cytotoxicity receptors of natural killer cells in cancer and infection. Trends Immunol 2013; 34: 182-91.

14. Bhat R and Rommelaere J. NK-cell-dependent killing of colon carcinoma cells is mediated by natural cytotoxicity receptors (NCRs) and stimulated by parvovirus infection of target cells. BMC Cancer 2013; 13: 367.

15. Raulet DH, Gasser S, Gowen BG, Deng W and Jung H. Regulation of ligands for the NKG2D activating receptor. Annu Rev Immunol 2013; 31: 413-41.

16. Zafirova B, Wensveen FM, Gulin M and Polic B. Regulation of immune cell function and differentiation by the NKG2D receptor. Cell Mol Life Sci 2011; 68: 3519-29.

17. de Andrade LF, Smyth MJ and Martinet L. DNAM-1 control of natural killer cells functions through nectin and nectin-like proteins. Immunol Cell Biol 2013;

18. Tahara-Hanaoka S, Miyamoto A, Hara A, Honda S, Shibuya K and Shibuya A. Identification and characterization of murine DNAM-1 (CD226) and its poliovirus receptor family ligands. Biochem Biophys Res Commun 2005; 329: 996-1000.

19. El-Sherbiny YM, Meade JL, Holmes TD, McGonagle D, Mackie SL, Morgan AW, Cook G, Feyler S, Richards SJ, Davies FE, Morgan GJ and Cook GP. The requirement for DNAM-1, NKG2D, and NKp46 in the natural killer cell-mediated killing of myeloma cells. Cancer Res 2007; 67: 8444-9.

20. Claus M, Meinke S, Bhat R and Watzl C. Regulation of NK cell activity by 2B4, NTB-A and CRACC. Front Biosci

2008; 13: 956-65.

21. Chan CJ, Smyth MJ and Martinet L. Molecular mechanisms of natural killer cell activation in response to cellular stress. Cell Death Differ 2014; 21: 5-14.

22. Bryceson YT, March ME, Ljunggren HG and Long EO. Activation, coactivation, and costimulation of resting human natural killer cells. Immunol Rev 2006; 214: 73-91.

23. Lam RA, Chwee JY, Le Bert N, Sauer M, Pogge von Strandmann E and Gasser S. Regulation of self-ligands for activating natural killer cell receptors. Ann Med 2013; 45: 384-94.

3. Expression characteristics of complement system related genes in patients with AMI and SAP

The complement system is an innate cytotoxic host defense system that normally functions to eliminate foreign pathogens and self-particles and can be activated via three different mechanisms, i.e., by classical, lectin or alternative pathways. The initiation of each pathway eventually results in the formation of terminal C5b-9 complex-the MAC (membrane attack complex) responsible mostly for cell lysis. Activation of the complement system also results in the productions of numerous effector molecules with potent biological activities: complement-mediated opsonization and phagocytosis by C3b, C4b and ic3b recognized by complement receptors, and anaphylatoxin production through C3a, C4a and C5a [1].

According to clinical research results, monomeric c-reactive protein (mCRP), myocardial necrosis and apoptotic cells might serve as potent activators of the complement system [2-4]. However, the extent of activation in the complement system with different forms of coronary atherosclerosis diseases (CAD) has not been fully elucidated, especially, few studies have been performed during stable angina pectoris (SAP), mostly with controversial results [5-8].

The complement system is composed of more than 30 different proteins, including complement components, receptors and regulators, which act in concern to generate immunoprotective and proinflammatory products. In clinical practice, it's hard to detect the levels of all proteins in the complement system currently. Therefore, in the present study, human microarray analysis was used to systematically examine the mRNA expressions of the complement components, receptors and regulators in peripheral blood mononuclear cells (PBMCs) isolated from acute myocardial infarction (AMI), SAP patients and the controls. We designed this *in vitro* study to investigate the changes in the function of complement system in patients with AMI and SA.

Results

Gene Expression of Complement Components
We detected mRNA expressions of complement early components including C1qα,

C1qβ, C1qγ, C1r, C1s, C2, C3, C4b, Factor B, Factor D, Factor P, MBL, MASP1, and MASP2 in PBMCs from three groups of patients (Figure 12-3-1A). In PBMCs from the three groups, expression levels of the genes encoding C1qα, C1qβ, C1qγ, C1r, Factor P and C1s were significantly different ($P<0.05$). In AMI, expression of C1qα ($P<0.05$), C1qβ, C1qγ, C1r and Factor P ($P<0.01$) was significantly up-regulated compared with SAP patients and controls, respectively, whereas C1s mRNA expression in AMI patients was down-regulated ($P<0.05$) compared with controls. Simultaneously, another three gene expressions (MBL, MASP1 and MASP2) had a lowest trend ($p>0.05$) in AMI among three groups. Between SAP and control group, there was no significant difference in mRNA expression.

Gene expressions of complement late components including C5, C6, C7, C8α, C8β, C8, and C9 in PBMCs from three groups of patients were examined (Figure 12-3-1B). In AMI patients, mRNA expression of C5 was significantly up-regulated ($P<0.01$) in comparison with SAP and control patients separately. In AMI patients, the gene expressions of C7, C8 and C9 were lowest among the three groups ($p>0.05$). There was also no significant difference of mRNA expression between SAP and the control group in late complement components.

Gene Expression of Complement Receptors

Were examined mRNA expression of complement receptors including CR1, CR2, C3aR, integrin αM, integrin αX, integrin β2, C5aR and CRIg in PBMCs from the three groups (Figure 12-3-2A). CR3 consists of integrin αM and integrin β2, and CR4 comprises integrin αX and integrin β2. In PBMCs from the three groups, expression of the genes encoding CR1, CR2, tegrin αM integrin αX, integrin β2, C5aR and CRIg was significantly different ($P<0.01$). In AMI patients, mRNA expression of genes CR1, integrin αM, integrin αX, integrin β2, C5aR and CRIg was significantly up-regulated compared with SAP patients and controls respectively ($P<0.05$). The mRNA expression of CR2 in both AMI and SAP patients was significantly down-regulated in comparison with the controls ($P<0.01$).

Gene Expression of Complement Regulators

Gene expression of complement regulators including C1 inhibitory factor(C1INH), C4b binding protein, α(C4bα), C4b binding protein, β(C4bβ), Factor I, Factor H, Factor H-related protein 1 (CFHR-1), CD46(MCP), CD55(DAF), vitronectin (VTN), clusterin (CLU) and CD59(MIRL)in PBMCs from the three groups was detected (Figure 12-3-2B). CD46, CD55 and CD59 mRNAs were significantly different among the three groups($P<0.01$). In PBMCs of AMI group, expression of the genes encoding CD46, CD55 and CD59 was significantly up-regulated compared apart with the other two groups ($P<0.01$). There was no significant gene expression difference between the SAP and control group in complement regulators either.

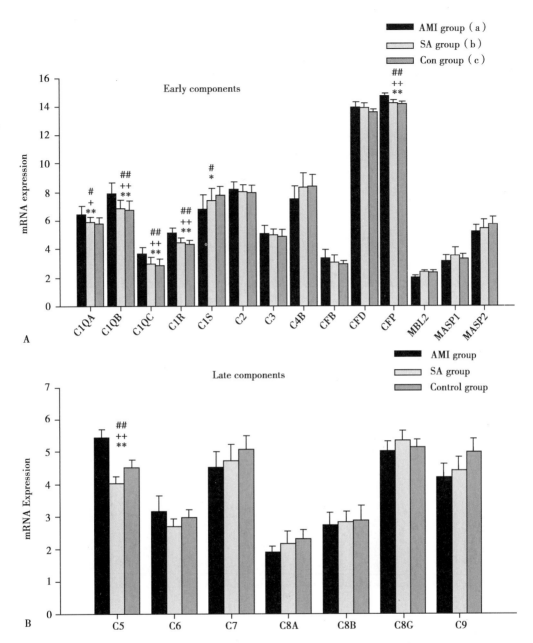

Figure 12-3-1　mRNA expression of complement early(A) and late(B)components in PBMCs from three groups.Three groups *P<0.05,**P<0.01. a v c $^{#}$P<0.05, $^{##}$P<0.01. a v b $^{+}$P<0.05,$^{++}$P<0.01. b v c $^{&}$P<0.05, $^{&&}$P<0.01. (Molecular Medicine Reports, 2016, 14(6): 5350)

In the present study, we examined early complement components of the three complement pathways and found that C1qα, C1qβ, C1qγ and C1r mRNAs were significantly up-regulated in AMI patients compared respectively with SAP patients and controls. The up-regulation of C1qα,C1qβ,C1qγ and C1r mRNAs suggested that the classical pathway, which is typically initiated by IgM or IgG-antibody/antigen immune complexes, was activated in AMI patients [9]. The alternative pathway is activated

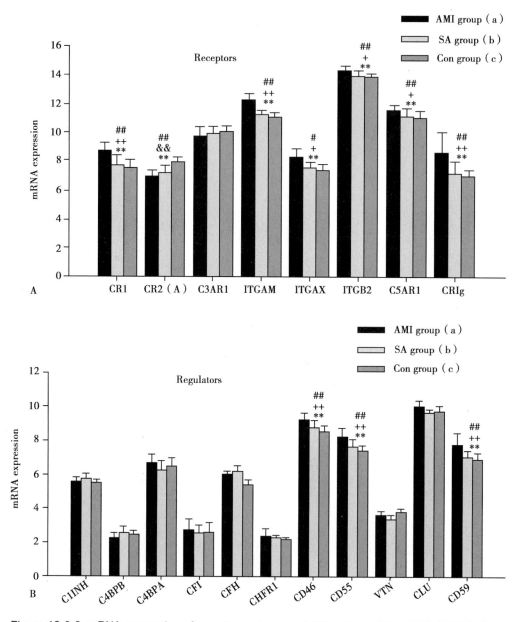

Figure 12-3-2. mRNA expression of complement receceports(A) and regulators(B) in PBMCs from three groups. Three groups *P<0.05, **P<0.01. a v c #P<0.05, ##P<0.01. a v b +P<0.05,++P<0.01. b v c &P<0.05, &&P<0.01. (Molecular Medicine Reports, 2016, 14(6): 5350)

mostly by "foreign surfaces", through the spontaneous hydrolysis of C3-C3b, and factor P plays an important role in the formation of C5 convertase. In our study, mRNA expression of factor P in the AMI group was significantly increased in comparison with the SAp and control groups, showing that the alternative pathway might also be activated. The activation of both the classical and alternative pathways in our study was consistent with the results from previous clinical studies [4,6,9]. When mannose-bind lectin (MBL) or Ficolin bind to carbohydrates on the surface of pathogens, the MBL-associated serine proteases (MASPs) are activated, then the lectin pathway is activated [10]. Previous studies had shown that people with MBL and MBL-associated MASPs deficiencies had immune dysfunctions and are susceptible to exotic pathogens [11-14]. Gene expression of MBL, MASP1 and MASP2 in AMI patients was the lowest among the three groups, therefore the downward of the three genes indicated the decline of the lectin pathway function in the AMI group. In SAP patients, the gene expression of early complement components had no significant difference compared with the controls, indicating that no initiation of any complement pathways was activated in SAP.

Three distinct pathways share a common terminal access to form C5b-9 complex (MAC), which forms a transmembrane pore in the target cells' membrane that causes cell lysis and death. C5b initiates the formation of MAC, which consists of C5b, C6, C7, C8, and multiple molecules of C9. In our study, we detected expression of seven genes of late complement components, five of which including C7, C8α, C8β, C8 and C9 mRNAs were the lowest in AMI patients, although there is no significant difference among the three groups. The declined gene expression of C7, C8 and C9 in AMI patients might lead to the obstacle of MAC formation.

We examined gene expression of eight complement receptors, and CR1, CR3, CR4, C5aR and CRIg mRNAs were highest in AMI among the three groups, suggesting the interactions between some complement effector molecules (C3b, C4b, ic3b, c3d, c3c) and their receptors were enhanced. The complement effectors played a role in opsonization and phagocytosis and promoted mobilization, migration and proliferation of leukocytes. The mRNA expression of CR2 both in AMI and SAP patients was significantly down-regulated in contrast to the controls. CR2 is a B cell membrane glycoprotein that plays a central role in B-cell activation, survival and proliferation. CR2 takes an important part in the recognition of foreign DNA from bacteria, viruses and other pathogens during host-immune responses [15,16]. In our study, gene expression of CR2 was significantly down-regulated in AMI and SAP groups, suggesting the immune dysfunction in B cells and might increase the risk of infections in both AMI and SAP patients.

Gene expression of eleven complement regulators was also detected in our study. The results showed that the mRNA expression of CD46, CD55 and CD59 was significantly up-regulated in the AMI group compared with the other two groups. CD46, known as a member cofactor protein, acts as a cofactor for factor I in the degradation of C3b and C4b, therefore inhibiting the convertase formation. CD55, also known as decay accelerating factor, accelerates the decay of C3 and C5 convertases. The complement receptor 1 (CR1/CD35) belongs to the regulators of complement activation protein family and displays both CD46 and CD55 activities [17]. CD59 can bind to C8 (αchain) and C9 during MAC complex formation and protects host cells from MAC-mediated lysis [18,19]. The all up-regulated gene expression of CD35, CD46, CD55 and CD59 in AMI patients suggested the inhibition of MAC-mediated cell lysis. The same as early components, there was no statistical difference of mRNA expression between SAP patients and controls in complement regulators, and our result was consistent with the conclusion from the studies of Yasuda and Kostner [7,8], who concluded that complement effector molecules were elevated in patients with AMI and unstable angina pectoris (UAP) but not in patients with SA.

During our present study, several early components of the classic pathway and the alternative pathway and complement receptors mRNAs were significantly up-regulated in AMI patients, suggesting the activation of the complement system. However, mRNAs expression of the formation of MAC was significantly decreased, suggesting the dysfunction of the complement system. In conclusion, in AMI patients the complement system was unbalanced and finally reduced the ability of MAC-induced cell lysis. In SAP patients, we only found CR2 mRNA significantly down-regulated compared with controls, suggesting that the complement system was almost in a balance and inactive state.

References

1. Széplaki G, Varga L, Füst G, Prohászka Z.Role of complement in the pathomechanism of atherosclerotic vascular diseases.Mol Immunol. 2009 Sep;46(14):2784-93. PMID:19501908

2. Christia P, Frangogiannis NG.Targeting inflammatory pathways in myocardial infarction.Eur J Clin Invest. 2013;43(9):986-95.

3. Cubedo J, Padró T, Badimon L.Coordinated proteomic signature changes in immune response and complement proteins in acute myocardial infarction: The implication of serum amyloid P-component. Int J Cardiol. 2013 15;168(6):5196-204.

4. Mihlan M, Blom AM, Kupreishvili K, et al.Monomeric C-reactive protein modulates classic complement activation on necrotic cells.FASEB J. 2011;25(12):4198-210.

5. Giasuddin AS, ElMahdawi JM, ElHassadi FM.Serum complement (C3, C4) levels in patients with acute myocardial infarction and angina pectoris.Bangladesh Med Res Counc Bull. 2007;33(3):98-102.

6. Iltumur K, Karabulut A, Toprak G, Toprak N.Complement activation in acute coronary syndromes.APMIS. 2005;113(3):167-74.

7. Kostner KM, Fahti RB, Case C, Hobson P, Tate J, Marwick TH.Inflammation, complement activation and endothelial function in stable and unstable coronary artery disease.Clin Chim Acta. 2006;365(1-2):129-34.

8. Yasuda M, Takeuchi K, Hiruma M, et al.The complement system in ischemic heart disease.Circulation. 1990;81(1):156-3

9. Horváth Z, Csuka D, Vargova K,et al.Elevated C1rC1sC1inh levels independently predict atherosclerotic coronary heart disease.Mol Immunol.2013;54(1):8-13.

10. Takahashi M, Mori S, Shigeta S, Fujita T. Role of MBL-associated serine protease (MASP) on activation of the

lectin complement pathway. Adv Exp Med Biol. 2007;598:93-104.

11. Pesonen E, Hallman M, Sarna S, et al.Mannose-binding lectin as a risk factor for acute coronary syndromes.Ann Med. 2009;41(8):591-8.

12. Koch A, Melbye M, Sørensen P, Homøe P, Madsen HO, Mølbak K, Hansen CH, Andersen LH, Hahn GW, Garred P. Acute respiratory tract infections and mannose-binding lectin insufficiency during early childhood. JAMA. 2001 Mar 14;285(10):1316-21.

13. Peterslund NA, Koch C, Jensenius JC, Thiel S. Association between deficiency of mannose-binding lectin and severe infections after chemotherapy. Lancet. 2001 Aug 25;358(9282):637-8.

14. Ali YM, Lynch NJ, Haleem KS, et al.The lectin pathway of complement activation is a critical component of the innate immune response to pneumococcal infection. PLoS Pathog. 2012;8(7):e1002793.

15. Low HZ, Hilbrans D, Schmidt-Wolf IG, Illges H.Enhanced CD21 expression and shedding in chronic lymphatic leukemia: a possible pathomechanism in disease progression.Int J Hematol. 2012;96(3):350-6.

16. Asokan R, Banda NK, Szakonyi G, Chen XS, Holers VM. Human complement receptor 2 (CR2/CD21) as a receptor for DNA: implications for its roles in the immune response and the pathogenesis of systemic lupus erythematosus (SLE).Mol Immunol. 2013;53(1-2):99-110.

17. Nuutila J, Jalava-Karvinen P, Hohenthal U,et al.Use of complement regulators, CD35, CD46, CD55, and CD59, on leukocytes as markers for diagnosis of viral and bacterial infections.Hum Immunol.2013;74(5):522-30..

18. Huang Y, Qiao F, Abagyan R, Hazard S, Tomlinson S. Defining the CD59-C9 binding interaction. J Biol Chem. 2006 Sep 15;281(37):27398-404.

19. Mayilyan KR. Complement genetics, deficiencies, and disease associations. Protein Cell. 2012;3(7):487-96.

4. Expression characteristics of cytokine related genes in patients with AMI and SAP

In the present study, human microarray analysis was used to systematically examine the mRNA expression of interferons (IFNs), interleukins (ILs), chemokines, tumor necrosis factors (TNFs) and associated receptors in peripheral blood mononuclear cells (PBMCs) isolated from AMI, SAP patients and controls. We designed this *in-vitro* study to investigate the differential gene expression of CK and analyzed the impacts on immune functions in the patients with AMI and SA.

Results

IFN mRNA expression levels

Expression of fifteen genes was detected in PBMCs from the three groups (Figure 12-4-1), including type I IFN, its receptors (IFNαR1, IFNαR2), type II IFN and its receptors (IFNγR1, IFNγR2). Type I IFNs consist of IFNα2, IFNα4, IFNα5, IFNα6, IFNα16, IFNα21, IFNβ1, IFNε, IFNκ, and IFNω1. PBMCs obtained from AMI patients demonstrated high mRNA expression levels. In the AMI group, IFNα2, IFNαR1, IFNαR2, IFNγR1, and IFNγR2 mRNA expressions were significantly up-regulated

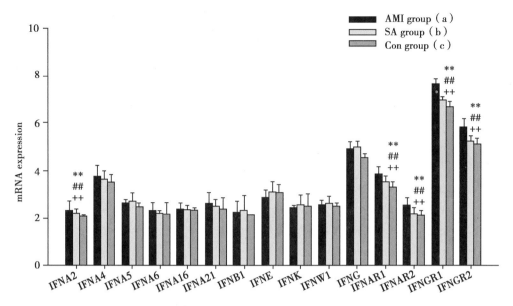

Figure 12-4-1 IFN mRNA expression levels Comparison within three groups: *P<0.05, **P<0.01; AMI vs. Control: #P<0.05; ##P<0.01; AMI vs. SA: +P<0.05, ++P<0.01; SA vs. Control: &P<0.05, &&P<0.01. (International Journal Of Clinical And Experimental Medicine,2015,8(10):18082-18089)

(P<0.01) than the SAP and control groups. Between the SAP and control groups, there was no significant difference in mRNA expression of the fifteen genes.

IL mRNA expression levels

The expression of fourteen IL gene of PBMCs from the three groups was examined (Figure 12-4-2), including IL1β, IL2, IL4, IL6, IL7, IL10, IL12A, IL15, IL16, IL17A, IL17F, IL18, IL22, and IL23A. In the AMI group, IL1β, IL2, IL16, and IL18 mRNAs were significantly up-regulated, while IL4 was significantly down-regulated compared with controls (P<0.05). Between the AMI and SAP groups, IL1β, IL16 and IL18 mRNAs in AMI patients were significantly up-regulated (P<0.01). However, there was no significant difference between the SAP group and the controls.

Chemokine mRNA expression

The comparison of gene expressions of chemokines and associated receptors in PBMCs from the three groups were shown in Figure 12-4-3. Fifteen gene expressions were detected, including CXC family and related receptors, CC family and associated receptors. In the AMI group, Cxcl5, Cxcl8, and CxcR1 mRNA expressions were significantly up-regulated (P<0.05), Cxcl1, Cxcl2, Cxcl6, CxcR2, and CxcR4 mRNA expressions were significantly up-regulated (P<0.01), while Ccl5, Ccl24, Ccl28 and CcR5 mRNA expressions were significantly downregulated (P<0.01) compared with controls. Compared with the SAP group, Cxcl1, Cxcl2, Cxcl6, CxcR2, and CxcR4 mRNA expressions in the AMI group were significantly up-regulated (P<0.01), and Ccl5, Ccl24,

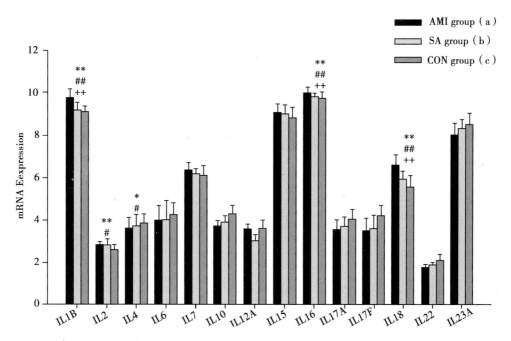

Figure 12-4-2　IL mRNA expression levels Comparison within three groups: *P<0.05, **P<0.01; AMI vs. Control: #P<0.05; ##P<0.01; AMI vs. SA: +P<0.05, ++P<0.01; SA vs. Control: &P<0.05, &&P<0.01. (International Journal Of Clinical And Experimental Medicine,2015,8(10):18082-18089)

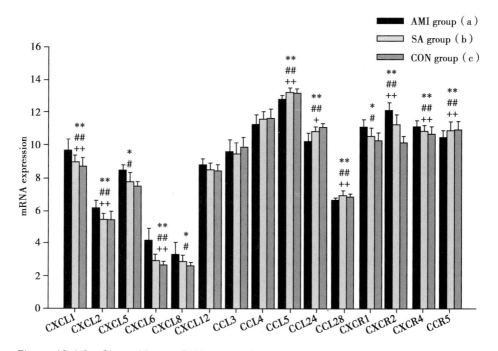

Figure 12-4-3　Chemokines mRNA expression levels Comparison within three groups: *P<0.05, **P<0.01; AMI vs. Control: #P<0.05; ##P<0.01; AMI vs. SA: +P<0.05, ++P<0.01; SA vs. Control: &P<0.05, &&P<0.01. (International Journal Of Clinical And Experimental Medicine,2015,8(10):18082-18089)

Ccl28, and CcR5 were significantly down-regulated (P<0.05). Between the SAP and control groups, there was no statistical difference in chemokines mRNA expression.

The TNF superfamily and TNF receptors superfamily mRNA expression levels

Fourteen mRNA expressions of the TNF superfamily genes (Figure 12-4-4A) and fifteen mRNA expressions of TNF receptors (Figure 12-4-4B) were detected in PBMCs

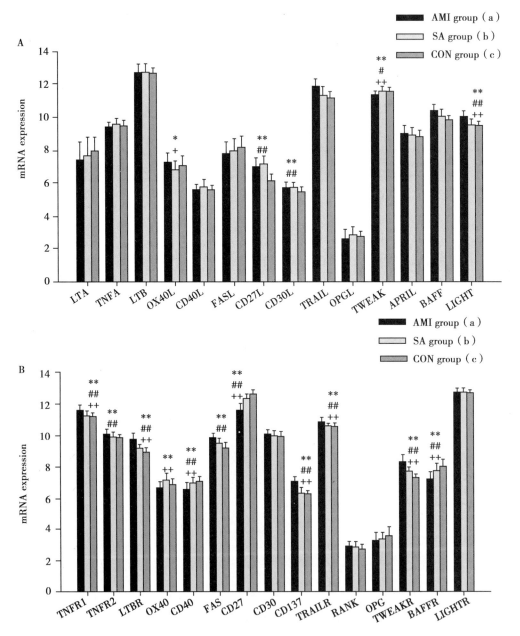

Figure 12-4-4   mRNA expressions of TNF (A) and associated receptors (B).Comparison within three groups: *P<0.05, **P<0.01; AMI vs. Control: #P<0.05; ##P<0.01; AMI vs. SA: +P<0.05, ++P<0.01; SA vs. Control: &P<0.05, &&P<0.01. (International Journal Of Clinical And Experimental Medicine,2015,8(10):18082-18089)

from the three groups. Compared with the control group, CD27L, CD30L, LIGHT, TNFR1, TNFR2, LT-βR, Fas, CD137, TRAILR, and TWEAKR mRNAs in the AMI patients were significantly up-regulated (P<0.01), while TWEAK, CD27, CD40 and BAFFR expressions were significantly down-regulated (P<0.05). Between the AMI and SAP groups, OX40L, LIGHT, TNFR1, LT-βR, CD137, TRAILR, and TWEAKR mRNAs in the AMI patients were significantly up-regulated (P<0.05), while OX40, TWEAK, CD40, CD27, and BAFFR mRNAs were significantly down-regulated (P<0.01). However, there was no significant difference between the SAP and control groups in mRNA expression of either TNF or TNF receptors.

IFNs are classified into two major groups: type Ⅰ and type Ⅱ. Type I IFNs include IFNα, IFNβ, IFNε, IFNω and IFNκ. Type Ⅰ IFNs use a heterodimeric receptor composed of the IFNAR1 and IFNAR2 chains, whereas type Ⅱ IFNs use a receptor formed by IFNGR1 and IFNGR2 [1]. IFNs possess anti-virus and immunomodulatory effects via JAK/STAT signaling pathway after binding to corresponding receptors[2]. Researchers found that IFNs play important roles in activation, differentiation and maturation of T lymphocytes and macrophages. The IFNs promoted expressions of MHC-Ⅰ and MHC-Ⅱ molecules on the surfaces of macrophages and activated cytotoxicity against pathogens [3,4]. It was reported that both human and animal IFN receptor deficiency models were prone to various kinds of infections [5,6]. The specific immune response to virus infections and autoimmune diseases was the detection of gene expressions of type I IFN in PBMC [7]. In the present study, gene expressions of IFNα2 and all IFN receptors were significantly up-regulated in the AMI patients, and no patients had the histories of tumors or autoimmune diseases, which indicate potential infections (especially by viruses) in the AMI patients and the enhanced activation and mobilization of T cells and macrophages. However, there was no significant difference between the SAP group and controls in the expression of IFNs.

Th precursor cells may be differentiated into Th1 or Th2 cells [8]. Th1 cells achieve cellular immunity mainly by secreting IL2, IL12 and IFN-γ, while Th2 cells produce IL4, IL5, IL6 and IL10 to promote the differentiation, maturation and proliferation of B lymphocytes and the generation of antibodies. The shift in Th1/Th2 balance leads to immunity dysfunction. Our results showed high mRNA expression of Th1 cytokines (IFN-γ and IL2) and low RNA expression of Th2 cytokines (IL4 and IL10) in the AMI patients, suggesting a shift towards Th1 dominance in the AMI patients. Th17 is also a major group of Th cells and the cytokines IL17A, IL17F, IL21 and IL22 secreted by Th17 cells can promote antigen-specific immunity crucial for the defense against bacterial and fungal invasion at the skin and mucosal surfaces [9,10]. Some researchers demonstrated that the Th1 cytokines suppress the differentiation of Th17 cells, and studies in mice showed that the differentiation of Th17 and Th1 cells was generally thought to be mutually exclusive[9]. In the present study, gene expressions of IL17A, IL17F, IL21 and

IL22 were down-regulated in AMI group, indicating the potential Th17 cell insufficiency in AMI patients. Thus, the unbalanced gene expressions of Th1, Th2 and Th17 cells suggested that an immune dysfunction in the AMI patients may exist.

Neutrophils are important components of the innate immunity. CXC chemokines and related receptors, taking part in immune responses by attracting neutrophils migrating to infected or injured parts, have strong effects on chemotaxis and activation of neutrophils [11,12]. In the study, CXCL1, CXCL2, CXCL5, CXCL6, CXC8, CXCR1, CXCR2, and CXCR4 mRNA expressions in AMI group were significantly up-regulated compared with the controls, suggesting the increased mobilization and recruitment of neutrophils in the AMI patients. However, there was no difference in CXC chemokine expressions between the SAP and control groups, indicating there was no chemotaxis and activation of neutrophils in the SAP patients.

The CC chemokines, CCL3 (MIP-1α), CCL4 (MIP-1β4) and CCL5 (RANTES), which are HIV inhibitory factors secreted by CD_8 T cells, have anti-virus effects by combining with CCR5 [13,14]. During chronic infections, virus-specific CD_8 T cell generated low level of cytokines and the cytotoxic ability of CD_8 T cells was decreased in CCL5 knockout mice [15]. Recent researches showed that CCR5 promoted NK cell proliferation and enhanced its cytotoxic ability [16], meanwhile CCR5 deficient individuals were susceptible to the virus [17,18]. As part of the innate immune system, CCL28 played antimicrobial activity independently [19,20]. In this study, the expression of CCL3, CCL4, CCL5, CCR5 and CCL28 was down-regulated in the AMI patients when compared with the controls, indicating that a reduced anti-virus ability and increased susceptibilities to external pathogens in AMI patients may exist. However, there was no significant difference between SAP and the controls in chemokine expression.

The TNF/TNFR superfamily genes play a significant role in immune responses [21]. Fas, an apoptosis factor, could result in direct apoptosis of B lymphocytes [22]. TNFR1 ligand pathway could induce activation-induced T cell death and aberrant T cell activation in stable heart transplantation patients [23]. Tsakiri reported that the TNFR2 signals could inhibit the activation of Treg cells in mice [24]. CD137, the co-stimulatory molecules of T lymphocytes, can inhibit the activities of both CD_4 T lymphocytes and NK cells [25,26]. In the present study, compared with the controls, FAS, TNFR1, TNFR2, and CD137 mRNA expressions were significantly up-regulated in the AMI patients, showing the decreased or suppressed activities of immune cells, thus an unbalanced immune function in AMI patients.

Wealth of data implicated TWEAK as a disease-susceptibility gene for a humoral immunodeficiency, and a low expression of TWEAK may lead to antibody deficiency [27]. The CD40/CD40L ligand interaction was important for promoting T-cell-mediated immunity, and people with CD40 deficiency were always accompanied by both dysfunction of T cell immunity and functional defects of dendritic cells [28]. OX40 and

CD27 are co-stimulatory factors of T lymphocytes, which regulate the proliferation and survival of CD_4 and CD_8T lymphocytes by binding to ligands, which are expressed by dendritic cells. So OX40 and CD27 deficiency would lead to dysfunction of T cells immunity [29,30]. It was reported that BAFFR deficiency could lead to decrement of transitional and follicular B lymphocytes in mice [31]. In our current study, TWEAK, CD40, OX40, CD27, and BAFFR mRNA expressions in the AMI group were significantly down-regulated while compared with SAP and/or control groups, which revealed that a dysfunction of immune system may exist in the AMI patients. There was no significant difference between the SAP and control group in SFPs expression.

Taken together, the present study indicated that the dysfunction of immune system in the AMI patients may be an internal factor of AMI pathogenesis, and infections, acting as a trigger in the process of AMI could be an external cause. The combined effects of internal and external factors may lead to myocardial infarction. However, no activation of CK network was observed in the SAP patients, showing the significant differences of immune functions between the AMI and SAP patients.

(published: Int J Clin Exp Med 2015;8(10):18082-18089)

References

1. Abbas AK, Lichtman AH. Cellular and molecular immunology. 5th ed. Philadelphia: W.B. Saunders company; 2005.

2. Claudinon J, Monier MN, Lamaze C. Interfering with interferon receptor sorting and trafficking: impact on signaling. Biochimie 2007; 89: 735-43.

3. Schroecksnadel K, Frick B, Winkler C, Fuchs D. Crucial role of interferon-gamma and stimulated macrophages in cardiovascular disease. Current vascular pharmacology 2006; 4: 205-13.

4. Foster GR, Masri SH, David R, Jones M, Datta A, Lombardi G et al. IFN-alpha subtypes differentially affect human T cell motility. Journal of immunology (Baltimore, Md.: 1950) 2004; 173: 1663-70.

5. Marazzi MG, Chapgier A, Defilippi AC, Pistoia V, Mangini S, Savioli C et al. Disseminated Mycobacterium scrofulaceum infection in a child with interferon-gamma receptor 1 deficiency. International journal of infectious diseases: IJID: official publication of the International Society for Infectious Diseases 2010; 14: e167-70.

6. van den Broek MF, Muller U, Huang S, Zinkernagel RM, Aguet M. Immune defence in mice lacking type I and/or type II interferon receptors. Immunological reviews 1995; 148: 5-18.

7. Kyogoku C, Smiljanovic B, Grun JR, Biesen R, Schulte-Wrede U, Haupl T et al. Cell-specific type I IFN signatures in autoimmunity and viral infection: what makes the difference? PloS one 2013; 8: e83776.

8. Constant SL, Bottomly K. Induction of Th1 and Th2 CD_4 T cell responses: the alternative approaches. Annual review of immunology 1997; 15: 297-322.

9. Zuniga LA, Jain R, Haines C, Cua DJ. Th17 cell development: from the cradle to the grave. Immunological reviews 2013; 252: 78-88.

10. Kolls JK, Khader SA. The role of Th17 cytokines in primary mucosal immunity. Cytokine & growth factor reviews

2010; 21: 443-8.

11. de Oliveira S, Reyes-Aldasoro CC, Candel S, Renshaw SA, Mulero V, Calado A. Cxcl8 (IL-8) mediates neutrophil recruitment and behavior in the zebrafish inflammatory response. Journal of immunology (Baltimore, Md.: 1950) 2013; 190: 4349-59.

12. Ritzman AM, Hughes-Hanks JM, Blaho VA, Wax LE, Mitchell WJ, Brown CR. The chemokine receptor CXCR2 ligand KC (CXCL1) mediates neutrophil recruitment and is critical for development of experimental Lyme arthritis and carditis. Infection and immunity 2010; 78: 4593-600.

13. Cocchi F, DeVico AL, Garzino-Demo A, Arya SK, Gallo RC, Lusso P. Identification of RANTES, MIP-1 alpha, and MIP-1 beta as the major HIV-suppressive factors produced by CD_8 T cells. Science (New York, N.Y.) 1995; 270: 1811-5.

14. Barrios CS, Castillo L, Zhi H, Giam CZ, Beilke MA. Human T cell leukaemia virus type 2 tax protein mediates CC-chemokine expression in peripheral blood mononuclear cells via the nuclear factor kappa B canonical pathway. Clinical and experimental immunology 2014; 175: 92-103.

15. Crawford A, Angelosanto JM, Nadwodny KL, Blackburn SD, Wherry EJ. A role for the chemokine RANTES in regulating CD_8 T cell responses during chronic viral infection. PLoS pathogens 2011; 7: e1002098.

16. Weiss ID, Shoham H, Wald O, Wald H, Beider K, Abraham M et al. Ccr5 deficiency regulates the proliferation and trafficking of natural killer cells under physiological conditions. Cytokine 2011; 54: 249-57.

17. Lim JK, McDermott DH, Lisco A, Foster GA, Krysztof D, Follmann D et al. CCR5 deficiency is a risk factor for early clinical manifestations of West Nile virus infection but not for viral transmission. The Journal of infectious diseases 2010; 201: 178-85.

18. Kohlmeier JE, Miller SC, Smith J, Lu B, Gerard C, Cookenham T et al. The chemokine receptor CCR5 plays a key role in the early memory CD_8 T cell response to respiratory virus infections. Immunity 2008; 29: 101-13.

19. Liu B, Wilson E. The antimicrobial activity of CCL28 is dependent on C-terminal positively-charged amino acids. European journal of immunology 2010; 40: 186-96.

20. Berri M, Virlogeux-Payant I, Chevaleyre C, Melo S, Zanello G, Salmon H et al. CCL28 involvement in mucosal tissues protection as a chemokine and as an antibacterial peptide. Developmental and comparative immunology 2014; 44: 286-90.

21. Matusik P, Guzik B, Weber C, Guzik TJ. Do we know enough about the immune pathogenesis of acute coronary syndromes to improve clinical practice? Thrombosis and haemostasis 2012; 108: 443-56.

22. Aggarwal BB, Gupta SC, Kim JH. Historical perspectives on tumor necrosis factor and its superfamily: 25 years later, a golden journey. Blood 2012; 119: 651-65.

23. Ankersmit HJ, Moser B, Zuckermann A, Roth G, Taghavi S, Brunner M et al. Activation-induced T cell death, and aberrant T cell activation via TNFR1 and CD95-CD95 ligand pathway in stable cardiac transplant recipients. Clinical and experimental immunology 2002; 128: 175-80.

24. Tsakiri N, Papadopoulos D, Denis MC, Mitsikostas DD, Kollias G. TNFR2 on non-haematopoietic cells is required for Foxp3+ Treg-cell function and disease suppression in EAE. European journal of immunology 2012; 42: 403-12.

25. Myers LM, Vella AT. Interfacing T-cell effector and regulatory function through CD137 (4-1BB) co-stimulation. Trends in immunology 2005; 26: 440-6.

26. Baessler T, Charton JE, Schmiedel BJ, Grunebach F, Krusch M, Wacker A et al. CD137 ligand mediates opposite effects in human and mouse NK cells and impairs NK-cell reactivity against human acute myeloid leukemia cells. Blood 2010; 115: 3058-69.

27. Wang HY, Ma CA, Zhao Y, Fan X, Zhou Q, Edmonds P et al. Antibody deficiency associated with an inherited autosomal dominant mutation in TWEAK. Proceedings of the National Academy of Sciences of the United States of America 2013; 110: 5127-32.

28. Fontana S, Moratto D, Mangal S, De Francesco M, Vermi W, Ferrari S et al. Functional defects of dendritic cells in patients with CD40 deficiency. Blood 2003; 102: 4099-106.

29. Locksley RM, Killeen N, Lenardo MJ. The TNF and TNF receptor superfamilies: integrating mammalian biology. Cell 2001; 104: 487-501.

30. Croft M, So T, Duan W, Soroosh P. The significance of OX40 and OX40L to T-cell biology and immune disease. Immunological reviews 2009; 229: 173-91.

31. Yan M, Brady JR, Chan B, Lee WP, Hsu B, Harless S et al. Identification of a novel receptor for B lymphocyte stimulator that is mutated in a mouse strain with severe B cell deficiency. Current biology: CB 2001; 11: 1547-52.

5. Expression characteristics of T cell related genes in AMI and SAP patients

T cells are key components of the adaptive immune system and plenty of data from human beings and mice suggest an essential role for T-cell-mediated immunity in atherosclerosis.[1-3] T cells can be divided into helper T cells (T helper cells, Th), cytotoxic T cells (cytotoxic T cell, CTL) and regulatory T cells (regulatory T cell, Treg). Various subsets of T cells can be found in the plaque rupture of coronary vessels, [4-6] and a number of animal models show that different subsets of T cells can drive or dampen inflammatory processes [7-9], but some results were controversial, for example, CTL and the balance of Th17/Treg subsets.[6,10-13] So quite a few issues on various T cell subset functions in humans still need to be uncovered especially in different stages of CAD, among which the acute myocardial infarction (AMI) and stable angina pectoris (SA) are most common cases.[14-15]

In the present study, we examined the expression of T cell related genes involved in T cell antigen recognition, activation and subset functions using human cDNA microarray analysis to identify gene expression differences in T cells in PBMCs isolated from AMI, SAP patients and controls. We designed this *in vitro* study to investigate the differential gene expression of T cell activation and functions of the subsets and then analyze the differences on cellular immunity in patients with AMI and SAP.

Results

Expression of genes related to T cell receptor (TCR) antigen recognition
Expression of 13 genes related to TCR antigen recognition in patients with AMI,

SAP and the control group was detected (Figure 12-5-1). Expression of 12 related genes in AMI was down-regulated compared to the SAP and control groups, and the genes encoding TCRA,TRB,TCRG,TCRZ,CD3D, CD3E,CD3G, CD8A and CD8B were significantly down-regulated (P<0.05) compared to the SAP patients and controls. Compared with controls, CD_4 mRNA in AMI was significantly down-regulated (P<0.05), and TCRIM expression in AMI group was significantly lower than that of SAP group (P<0.01). The TCR related genes in the SAP and control groups showed no significant difference.

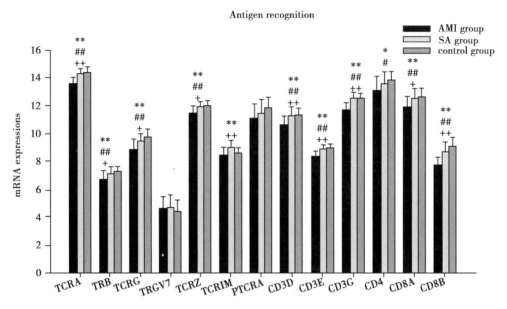

Figure 12-5-1   Expression of genes related to antigen recognition in T cell activation in PBMCs from three groups Three groups: *P<0.05; **P<0.01. a v c: #P<0.05; ##P<0.01. b v c:&P<0.05;&&P<0.01. a v b: +P<0.05; ++P<0.01. (International Journal Of Clinical And Experimental Medicine,2015,8(7):10875-10884)

Expression of genes related to co-stimulators and regulators of T cell activation

Expression of 16 genes related to co-stimulators and regulators of T cell activation in PBMCs from patients with AMI SAP and the control group was examined (Figure 12-5-2). In the AMI patients, 15 genes were lower and 8 encoding CD28, ICOS, B7-H2, CD2, CD40, LCK, FYN and LAT were significantly lower than the other two groups (P<0.05). MALT1 expression in AMI group was significantly lower than in controls (P<0.05). Between the SAP and control groups, there was no significant difference in T cell activation related expressions.

Expression of genes related to CTL

The results showed that the expression of 11 genes related to CTL in patients with AMI and SAP and the control group was detected (Figure 12-5-3A). In PBMCs from the three groups, all the 11 genes in AMI group were down-regulated, including the genes encoding GZMK, GZMM, PRF1 and CASP8 (P<0.05). Compared with SAP patients and

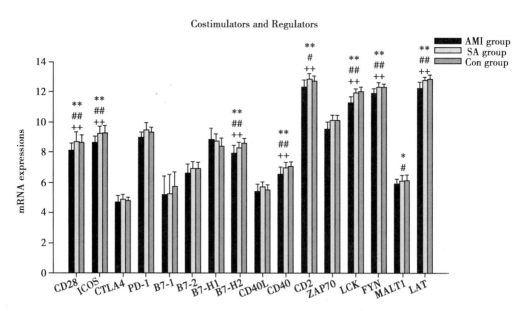

Figure 12-5-2   Expression of genes related to T cell receptors and regulators in T cell activation in PBMCs from three groups Three groups: *P<0.05; **P<0.01. a v c: #P<0.05; ##P<0.01. b v c:&P<0.05;&&P<0.01. a v b: +P<0.05; ++P<0.01. (International Journal Of Clinical And Experimental Medicine,2015,8(7):10875-10884)

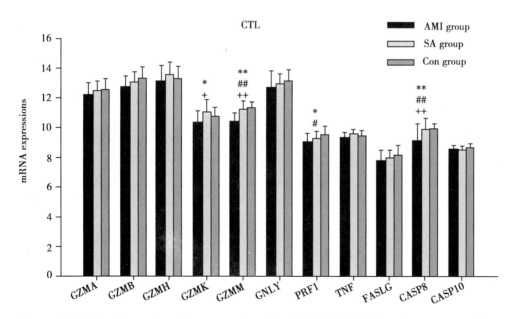

Figure 12-5-3A   Expression of genes related to CTL in PBMCs from three groups. Three groups:*P<0.05;**P<0.01.a v c: #P<0.05; ##P<0.01. b v c:&P<0.05;&&P<0.01. a v b: +P<0.05; ++P<0.01. (International Journal Of Clinical And Experimental Medicine, 2015, 8 (7): 10875-10884)

controls, mRNA expression of GZMM and CASP8 in AMI patients was significantly down-regulated (P<0.05). Compared with controls, PRF1 mRNA in the AMI group was significantly down-regulated (P<0.05), and GZMK expression in the AMI group was significantly lower than in SAP group (P<0.01). Between the SAP and control groups, there was no statistically significant difference in CTL related mRNA expression.

Expression of genes related to Th1/Th2

The results showed that mRNA expression of 15 genes related to Th1/Th2, including cytokines, transcription factors and chemokine receptors in PBMCs from AMI and SA and the control groups was detected (Figure 12-5-3B). Among the three groups, expression of the genes encoding IL1, IL2, IL18, CCR5, IL4, GATA3 and CRTH2 was significantly different (P<0.01). Compared with the controls, gene expression of IL1, IL2 and IL18 in the AMI group was significantly up-regulated (P<0.05), while CCR5, IL-4 and GATA3 mRNA expression was down-regulated (P<0.05). When compared with the SAP group, in the AMI patients, IL1 and IL18 genes were significantly higher (P<0.01), while CCR5, GATA3 and CRTH2 genes were significantly lower (P<0.01). Between the SAP and control groups, there was no significant difference in Th1/Th2 related mRNAs.

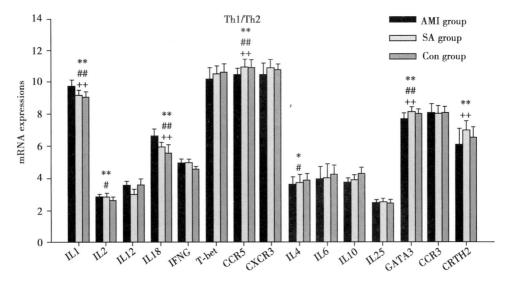

Figure 12-5-3B   Expression of genes related to Th1 and Th2 in PBMCs from three groups
Three groups: *P<0.05; **P<0.01. a v c: #P<0.05; ##P<0.01. b v c:&P<0.05;&&P<0.01. a v b: +P<0.05; ++P<0.01. (International Journal Of Clinical And Experimental Medicine, 2015, 8 (7): 10875-10884)

Expression of genes related toTh17/Tregs

mRNA expression of 13 genes related to Th17/Treg, including cytokines, transcription factors and chemokine receptors in PBMCs from AMI,SA and the control group was examined (Figure 12-5-3C). In PBMCs from the three groups, expression of

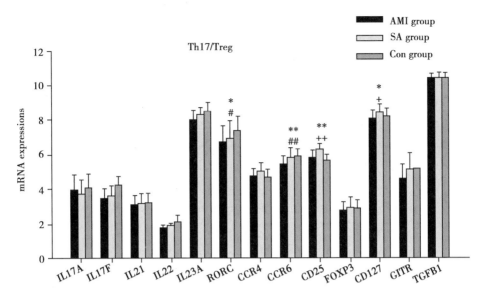

Figure 12-5-3C　Expression of genes related to Th17 and Treg in PBMCs from three groups
Three groups: *P<0.05; **P<0.01. a v c: #P<0.05; ##P<0.01. b v c: &P<0.05; &&P<0.01. a v b: +P< 0.05;
++P<0.01. (International Journal Of Clinical And Experimental Medicine, 2015, 8 (7): 10875-10884)

genes including RORC, CCR6, CD25 and CD127 was significantly different (P<0.05). Gene expression of RORC and CCR6 in the AMI group was significantly down-regulated when compared with the controls (P<0.05). CD25 and CD127 mRNAs in AMI were significantly lower (P<0.01) than those in the SAP group. Between the SAP and control groups, there was no significant difference in Th17/Treg related mRNA expression.

Expression of genes related to TCR antigen recognition

TCR is a molecule found on the surface of T lymphocytes that is responsible for recognizing antigens bounded to major histocompatibility complex (MHC) molecules. The TCR is composed of alpha (α)/beta (β) or gamma (γ)/delta (δ) heterodimers. T cells require two signals to become fully activated. The first signal, which is antigen-specific, is provided through the TCR-CD_3 complex which interacts with peptide-MHC molecules on the membrane of antigen presenting cells (APC).[16,17] Meanwhile, this signal is enhanced by a specific co-receptor. On helper T cells, this co-receptor is CD_4, which is specific for MHC class Ⅱ. On cytotoxic T cells, the co-receptor is CD_8, which is specific for MHC class I.[18] In our present study, gene expression of TCRA, TRB, TCRG, TCRZ, CD3D, CD3E and CD3G was significantly lower in AMI group, showing the decreased ability of TCR antigen recognition. Meanwhile, the significantly down-regulated CD_4, CD8A and CD8B mRNAs suggested that the T cell co-activation signal was attenuated. Taken together, the first T cell activation signal was weakened in the AMI patients. Between the SAP and control groups, there was no significant TCR antigen recognition mRNAs difference, which revealed the different TCR antigen recognition activity in the

AMI and SAP patients.

Expression of genes related to co-stimulators and regulators of T cell activation

A second signal, the co-stimulatory signal for T cell activation, is antigen non-specific and is provided by the interaction between co-stimulatory molecules expressed on the membrane of APC and T cells. The important co-stimulatory receptors expressed by T cells are the molecules of the CD28 family,[19] including CD28, cytotoxic T-lymphocyte-associated antigen 4 (CTLA-4), inducible co-stimulator (ICOS) and program death-1 (PD-1), which play a critical role in controlling T cell activation, proliferation and tolerance. CD28 and ICOS are both activated receptors, while CTLA4 and PD-1 are inhibitory receptors. These receptors recognize the B7 family, comprising B7-1 (CD80), B7-2 (CD86), B7-H1 (CD274) and B7-H2 (ICOSL), which are typically expressed by the APC.[20] The CD40 ligand (CD40L)/CD40 pathway is also involved in co-stimulation of T cell activation.[21] In our present study, CD28, ICOS, B7-H2 and CD40 mRNAs were significantly lower in the AMI patients, demonstrating that the second T cell activation signal was blocked. When the TCR engages with the two activating signals, a series of regulators, including co-receptors, associated enzymes and specialized adaptor molecules are also involved in T cell activation. The binding of CD2 co-receptor with its ligand is a non-specific pathway for T cell activation.[22] Zeta-associated protein of 70 kDa (ZAP-70) is the key enzyme in early T cell enzymatic reaction signal.[23] The Src-family kinases, Lck and Fyn, are central to the initiation of TCR signaling pathways and influence T cell activation and differentiation.[24,25] Recent findings define MALT1 (mucosa-associated-lymphoid-tissue lymphoma-translocation gene 1) as a protein with proteolytic activity that controls T cell activation by regulating key molecules in TCR induced signaling pathways.[26] The adaptor protein LAT serves as an integration node for signaling pathways that drive T cell activation.[27] In our study, expression of the genes including LCK, FYN, MALT1 and LAT was significantly lower in the AMI patients than those in the control group, demonstrating that T cell activation signal was inhibited in the AMI patients. There was no significant gene expression difference in T cell activation between the SAP and controls, suggesting that the decreased ability of T cells activation only occurred in the stage of the AMI patients.

Expression of genes related to CTL

CTLs kill virus-infected cells and tumor cells, and play a critical role in immune protection. Specific CTL killing involves three steps including antigen recognition, activation and fatal attack.[28] CTL is activated by TCR and CD_8 binding (the first signal) and co-stimulatory molecules (the second signal). The cytoplasmic granules in CTLs contain proteins erforins and granzymes. When the CTLs bind to their targets, the contents of the granules are discharged by exocytosis.[29] Another way of CTLs killing is through the FasL expressed on CTL surface and the secretion of TNF-α. When CTLs recognize their targets, they bind with the Fas and TNF receptors on the surface of target cells and lead to their apoptosis through caspase signals.[30] The presence of CTL cells in atherosclerotic lesions is widely demonstrated but studies investigating their role in atherogenesis have yielded contradictory results.[6,10] In our study, all 11 genes related to CTL killing ability in AMI patients were down-regulated, especially GZMK, GZMM, PRF1 and CASP8 were significantly down-regulated while compared with the SAP and/ or controls. As mentioned before, the TCR antigen recognizing and two signals of T cell activation were weakened in the AMI patients. However, there was no significant difference in CTL related mRNA expression between the SAP and control groups. All the results suggested the significantly different CTLs killing ability in the stages of AMI and SA.

Expression of genes related to Th1/Th2

After stimulation by several cytokines, naive CD_4 T cells differentiate into effector T cells, such as the T helper type 1 (Th1), T helper type 2 (Th2), and T helper type 17 (Th17) lineages.[31] Th1 cells achieve cellular immunity mainly by secreting IL1, IL2, IL12, IL18 and IFN-γ. T-bet is a Th1 transcription factor for regulating Th1 development,[32] and CCR5 and CXCR3 are specific Th1 lymphocytes chemokine receptors.[33,34] Th2 cells produce IL4, IL5, IL6, IL10 and IL25 to activate B lymphocytes and generate antibodies. GATA3 is the Th2 specific transcription factor, and CCR3 together with CRTH2 are chemokine receptors of Th2.[35-37] The shift in Th1/Th2 balance leads to immunity dysfunction. Our results showed in AMI patients the high mRNA expression of Th1 cytokines (IL1,IL2 and IL18) and low RNA expression of Th2 cytokines, transcription factor and chemokine receptors (IL4, GATA3 and CRTH2), suggesting a shift towards Th1 dominance in AMI. And this result is consistent with the experiments of Soltesz and Zhang.[38,39]

Th17 cells mainly produce cytokines IL17A, IL17F, IL21 and IL22, and have been observed in atherosclerotic plaques both in humans and animals.[40] Th17 cells can promote antigen-specific immunity crucial for the defense against bacterial and fungal invasion at the skin and mucosal surfaces.[41,42] RORC is the specific transcription factor of Th17,[43] and CCR4 and CCR6 are chemokine receptors of Th17.[44,45] It has been demonstrated that the Th1 cytokines suppress the differentiation of Th17 cells, and studies in mice showed that the differentiation of Th17 and Th1 cells is generally thought to be mutually exclusive.[41] In our present study, in AMI group gene expressions of IL17A, IL17F, IL21, IL22, IL23A, RORC, CCR4 and CCR6 were down-regulated, especially RORC and CCR6 were significantly down-regulated, while no significant difference was observed between the SAP and controls, which indicated the potential insufficiency of Th17 activity in the stage of AMI.

Tregs that possess anti-inflammatory properties have also been reported in atherosclerotic plaques [10,11]. Tregs are a minor subpopulation of T lymphocytes that maintain self-tolerance to autoantigens and suppress the activity of proatherogenic effector T cells taking an atheroprotective effect.[46] CD25, FOXP3 and CD127 are the specific surface markers for Tregs.[47,48] In addition, other various surface markers such as CD_3,CTLA-4 and GITR are also involved in the function of Tregs.[49] Several cytokines (including IL-10 and TGF-β) secreted by Tregs can inhibit APC activity. [50] In our study, in the AMI group, the expression of CD25, FoxP3, CD127, GTIR and TGFB1 was lower, while CD25 and CD127 were significantly lower than the SAP group, suggesting the dysfunction of Tregs.

Nowadays several studies suggested the essential role of Th17/Treg imbalance in the destabilization of CAD, whereas the data from the patients with SAP were controversial [10-14]. In our present study, in the AMI group, gene expression of both Th17 and Tregs was down-regulated, showing the imbalance of Th17/Tregs in AMI stage. No significant Th17 and Tregs related gene expression differences were observed between the SAP and control groups, consistent with the results of Ammirati and Potekhina.[51,52] Thus, the unbalanced gene expression of Th1/Th2 and Th17/Tregs suggested the different T cells activity in the AMI and SA stages of CAD, and an immune impairmentonly exists in the AMI patients.

In the AMI group, the TCR antigen recognition, binding, as well as the co-stimulators and regulators of T cell activation related gene expression were all significantly down-regulated, showing the T cell activation was inhibited in the AMI patients. The lower expression of genes related to CTLs showed the decreased killing ability of CTLs in the stage of AMI. The significantly differential expression of cytokines, transcription factors and chemokine receptors related to T cell subsets suggested an enhanced immune response in Th1 but a weakened response in Th2, Th17 and Tregs. However, there was no statistical gene expression difference in T cell related genes between the SAP and control groups. Therefore, the significantly different T cell expressions in the AMI and SAP patients indicated the different cellular immunity in these two stages of CAD. The reduced T cell activation and the dysfunction of T cell subsets were observed in the AMI stage in our study. As a consequence, improving T cell mediated cellular immunity may be considered as a potential target for medical interventions in the patients with AMI.

(published: Int J Clin Exp Med 2015;8(7):10875-10884)

References

1. van Dijk RA, Duinisveld AJ, Schaapherder AF, Mulder-Stapel A, Hamming JF, Kuiper J, de Boer OJ, van der Wal AC, Kolodgie FD, Virmani R, Lindeman JH.A change in inflammatory footprint precedes plaque instability: a systematic evaluation of cellular aspects of the adaptive immune response in human atherosclerosis.J Am Heart Assoc2015;26;4(4).

2. Robertson AK, Hansson GK.T cells in atherogenesis: for better or for worse?Arterioscler Thromb Vasc Biol2006;26(11):2421-2432.

3. Businaro R, Tagliani A, Buttari B, Profumo E, Ippoliti F, Di Cristofano C, Capoano R, Salvati B, Riganò R.Cellular and molecular players in the atherosclerotic plaque progression.Ann N Y Acad Sci2012;1262:134-141.

4. Grivel JC, Ivanova O, Pinegina N, Blank PS, Shpektor A, Margolis LB, Vasilieva E.Activation of T lymphocytes in atherosclerotic plaques.Arterioscler Thromb Vasc Biol2011;31(12):2929-2937.

5. Tarun Dave, J. Ezhilan, Hardik Vasnawala, and Vinod Somani.Plaque regression and plaque stabilisation in cardiovascular diseases.Indian J Endocrinol Metab2013; 17(6): 983-989.

6. Kyaw T, Winship A, Tay C, Kanellakis P, Hosseini H, Cao A, Li P, Tipping P, Bobik A, Toh BH.Cytotoxic and proinflammatory CD_8 T lymphocytes promote development of vulnerable atherosclerotic plaques in apoE-deficient mice.Circulation 2013;127(9):1028-1039.

7. Ni M, Chen WQ, Zhang Y.Animal models and potential mechanisms of plaque destabilisation and disruption. Heart2009;95(17):1393-1398.

8. Johnson JL, Jackson CL.Atherosclerotic plaque rupture in the apolipoprotein E knockout mouse.Atheroscleros is2001;154(2):399-406.

9. Tian Ma, Qi Gao, Faliang Zhu, Chun Guo, Qun Wang,Fei Gao, and Lining Zhang.Th17 cells and IL-17 are involved in the disruption of vulnerable plaques triggered by short-term combination stimulation in apolipoprotein E-knockout mice.Cell Mol Immunol2013; 10(4): 338-348.

10. Zhou J, Dimayuga PC, Zhao X, Yano J, Lio WM, Trinidad P, Honjo T, Cercek B, Shah PK, Chyu KY.CD_8(+)CD25(+) T cells reduce atherosclerosis in apoE(−/−) mice.Biochem Biophys Res Commun 2014;443(3):864-70.

11. Mor A, Luboshits G, Planer D, Keren G, George J.Altered status of CD_4CD25+ regulatory T cells in patients with acute coronary syndromes.Eur. Heart J2006;27:2530-2537.

12. Li Q, Wang Y, Wang Y, Chen K, Zhou Q, Wei W, Wang Y.Treg/Th17 ratio acts as a novel indicator for acute coronary syndrome. Cell Biochem Biophys 2014;70(2):1489-1498.

13. Zhang L, Wang T, Wang XQ, Du RZ, Zhang KN, Liu XG, Ma DX, Yu S, Su GH, Li ZH, Guan YQ, Du NL.Elevated frequencies of circulating Th22 cell in addition to Th17 cell and Th17/Th1 cell in patients with acute coronary syndrome. PLoS One 2013;8(12):e71466.

14. Aukrust P, Otterdal K, Yndestad A, Sandberg WJ, Smith C, Ueland T, Øie E, Damås JK, Gullestad L, Halvorsen B. The complex role of T-cell-based immunity in atherosclerosis. Curr Atheroscler Rep 2008; 10: 236-243.

15. Matusik P, Guzik B, Weber C, Guzik TJ. Do we know enough about the immune pathogenesis of acute coronary syndromes to improve clinical practice? Thromb Haemost 2012; 108: 443-456.

16. Guy CS, Vignali DA. Organization of proximal signal initiation at the TCR:CD_3 complex. Immunol Rev 2009; 232: 7-21.

17. Zehn D, King C, Bevan MJ,Palmer E. TCR signaling requirements for activating T cells and for generating memory. Cell Mol Life Sci 2012; 69: 1565-1575.

18. König R. Interactions between MHC molecules and co-receptors of the TCR. Curr Opin Immunol 2002; 14: 75-83.

19. Riley JL, June CH. The CD28 family: a T-cell rheostat for therapeutic control of T-cell activation. Blood 2005; 105: 13-21.

20. Hansen JD, Pasquier LD, Lefranc M-P,Lopez V, Benmansour A, Boudinot P.The B7 family of immunoregulatory receptors: a comparative and evolutionary perspective. Mol Immunol 2009; 46: 457-472.

21. Howland KC, Ausubel LJ, London CA, Abbas AK. The roles of CD28 and CD40 ligand in T cell activation and tolerance. J Immunol 2000; 164: 4465-4470.

22. Sigrid SS, Kristine M, Torunn B,Aandahl EM, Taskén K. T-cell co-stimulation through the CD2 and CD28 co-receptors induces distinct signalling responses. Biochem J 2014; 460: 399-410.

23. Lin H, Martelli MP, Bierer BE. The involvement of the proto-oncogene p120 c-Cbl and ZAP-70 in CD2-mediated T cell activation. Int Immunol 2001; 13: 13-22.

24. Salmond RJ, Filby A, Qureshi I, Caserta S, Zamoyska R. T-cell receptor proximal signaling via the Src-family kinases, Lck and Fyn, influences T-cell activation, differentiation, and tolerance. Immunol Rev 2009; 228: 9-22.

25. Palacios EH, Weiss A. Function of the Src-family kinases, Lck and Fyn, in T-cell development and activation. Oncogene 2004; 23: 7990-8000.

26. Thome M. Multifunctional roles for MALT1 in T-cell activation. Nat Rev Immunol 2008; 8: 495-500.

27. Bartelt RR, Houtman JCD. The adaptor protein LAT serves as an integration node for signaling pathways that drive T cell activation. Wiley Interdiscip Rev Syst Biol Med 2013; 5: 101-110.

28. Gadhamsetty S, Marée AFM, Beltman JB, de Boer RJ. A General Functional Response of Cytotoxic T Lymphocyte-Mediated Killing of Target Cells. Biophys J 2014; 106: 1780-1791.

29. Keefe D, Shi L, Feske S, Massol R, Navarro F, Kirchhausen T, Lieberman J. Perforin triggers a plasma membrane-repair response that facilitates CTL induction of apoptosis. Immunity 2005; 23: 249-262.

30. Berke G. The CTL's kiss of death. Cell 1995; 81: 9-12.

31. Constant SL, Bottomly K. Induction of Th1 and Th2 CD_4 T cell responses: the alternative approaches. Annu Rev Immunol 1997; 15: 297-322.

32. Vanaki E, Ataei M, Sanati MH, Mansouri P, Mahmoudi M, Zarei F, Jadali Z.Expression patterns of Th1/Th2 transcription factors in patients with guttate psoriasis. Acta Microbiol Immunol Hung 2013; 60: 163-174.

33. Gao P, Zhou XY, Yashiro-Ohtani Y, Yang YF, Sugimoto N, Ono S, Nakanishi T, Obika S, Imanishi T, Egawa T, Nagasawa T, Fujiwara H, Hamaoka T.The unique target specificity of a nonpeptide chemokine receptor antagonist: selective blockade of two Th1 chemokine receptors CCR5 and CXCR3. J Leukoc Biol 2003; 73: 273-280.

34. Loetscher P, Uguccioni M, Bordoli L, Baggiolini M, Moser B, Chizzolini C, Dayer JM. CCR5 is characteristic of Th1 lymphocytes. Nature 1998; 391: 344-345.

35. Wan YY. GATA3: a master of many trades in immune regulation. Trends Immunol 2014; 35: 233-242.

36. Sallusto F, Mackay CR, Lanzavecchia A. Selective expression of the eotaxin receptor CCR3 by human T helper 2 cells. Science 1997; 277: 2005-2007.

37. Nagata K, Hirai H. The second PGD_2 receptor CRTH2: structure, properties, and functions in leukocytes. Prostaglandins Leukot Essent Fatty Acids 2003; 69: 169-177.

38. Szodoray P, Timar O, Veres K, Der H, Szomjak E, Lakos G, Aleksza M, Nakken B, Szegedi G, Soltesz P.TH1/TH2 imbalance, measured by circulating and intracytoplasmic inflammatory cytokines--immunological alterations in acute coronary syndrome and stable coronary artery disease.Scand J Immunol2006;64(3):336-344.

39. Cheng X, Liao YH, Ge H, Li B, Zhang J, Yuan J, Wang M, Liu Y, Guo Z, Chen J, Zhang J, Zhang L.TH1/TH2 functional

imbalance after acute myocardial infarction: coronary arterial inflammation or myocardial inflammation.J Clin Immunol2005;25(3):246-253.

40. Eid RE, Rao DA, Zhou J, Lo SF, Ranjbaran H, Gallo A, Sokol SI, Pfau S, Pober JS, Tellides G.Interleukin-17 and interferon-gamma are produced concomitantly by human coronary artery-infiltrating T cells and act synergistically on vascular smooth muscle cells.Circulation2009; 119:1424-1432.

41. Zuniga LA, Jain R, Haines C, Cua DJ.Th17 cell development: from the cradle to the grave. Immunol Rev 2013; 252: 78-88.

42. Kolls JK, Khader SA. The role of Th17 cytokines in primary mucosal immunity. Cytokine Growth Factor Rev 2010; 21: 443-448.

43. Unutmaz D. RORC2: the master of human Th17 cell programming. Eur J Immunol 2009; 39: 1452-1455.

44. Wang C, Kang SG, Lee J, Sun Z, Kim CH. The roles of CCR6 in migration of Th17 cells and regulation of effector T-cell balance in the gut. Mucosal Immunol 2009; 2: 173-183.

45. Moriguchi K, Miyamoto K, Tanaka N, Yoshie O, Kusunoki S.The importance of CCR4 and CCR6 in experimental autoimmune encephalomyelitis. J Neuroimmunol 2013; 257: 53-58.

46. H. von Boehmer.Mechanisms of suppression by suppressor T cells.Nat. Immunol2005;6:338-344.

47. Klein S, Kretz CC, Krammer PH, Kuhn A. CD127low/- and FoxP3+ Expression Levels Characterize Different Regulatory T-Cell Populations in Human Peripheral Blood. J Invest Dermatol 2009; 130: 492-499.

48. Hall BM, Verma ND, Tran GT, Hodgkinson SJ.Distinct regulatory CD_4^+ T cell subsets; differences between naïve and antigen specific T regulatory cells. Curr Opin Immunol 2011; 23: 641-647.

49. Ephrem A, Epstein AL, Stephens GL,Thornton AM, Glass D, Shevach EM. Modulation of Treg cells/T effector function by GITR signaling is context-dependent. Eur J Immunol 2013; 43: 2421-2429.

50 Caridade M, Graca L, Ribeiro RM. Mechanisms underlying CD_4 Treg immune regulation in the adult: from experiments to models. Front Immunol2013; 4: 387.

51. Potekhina AV, Pylaeva E, Provatorov S, Ruleva N, Masenko, Noeva E, Krasnikova T, Arefieva T.Treg/Th17 balance in stable CAD patients with different stages of coronary atherosclerosis.Atherosclerosis2015;238(1):17-21.

52. Ammirati E, Cianflone D, Banfi M, Vecchio V, Palini A, De Metrio M, Marenzi G, Panciroli C, Tumminello G, Anzuini A, Palloshi A, Grigore L, Garlaschelli K, Tramontana S, Tavano D, Airoldi F, Manfredi AA, Catapano AL, Norata GD.Circulating $CD_4CD25hiCD127lo$ regulatory T-Cell levels do not reflect the extent or severity of carotid and coronary atherosclerosis.ArteriosclerThrombVasc Biol2010;30 (9):1832-1841.

6. Expression characteristics of B cell related genes in patients with AMI and SAP

The presence of B lymphocytes in inflammatory infiltration in humans [1,2] and mice models [3,4] has led to an urgent need for searching its role in atherosclerosis. However, the role of B cells in atherogenesis is still controversial. T-independent B cells (B1 cells) may be endowed with atheroprotective properties,[5,6] whereas T-dependent B cells (B2 cells) have proatherogenic potential. [7,8] B cell activation requires two signals. The first is the binding of antigens to the B cell antigen receptor (BCR), which is expressed on the surface of B cells. With a thymus-independent antigen, B cells can deliver the second signal by themselves. With a thymus-dependent antigen, the second signal comes from the interaction between T cells and B cells. [9] Broadly, B1 and B2 cells constitute the major two groups of B cells and can be considered a part of the innate and adaptive immune systems, respectively. [10] B1 cell is a minor part of B cells, producing natural antibodies to common microbial epitopes and self-determinants. B2 cell is considered as the conventional B lymphocytes requiring helper T cell signals to recognize specific antigens, produce and regulate antibody-mediated humoral immunity. [11,12]

In the present study, the expression of a wide range of B cell-related genes involved in B cell activation was examined. The human cDNA microarray analysis was used to detect the variations in gene expression in different stages of B cell activation and subsets in peripheral blood mononuclear cells (PBMCs) isolated from the AMI patients, stable angina (SA) patients and controls. We designed the *in-vitro* study to investigate the differential gene expression of B cells and analyzed the differences on humoral immunity in patients with AMI and SA.

Results

Expression of genes related to BCR

The results showed that expression of 22 genes related to BCR in patients with AMI, SAP and the controls was detected (Figure 12-6-1). In PBMCs from the three groups, expression of 15 genes encoding CD45, NFAM1, BTK, SYK, LYN, FCRL3, CD79A, CD79B, CD19, CD21, CD81, FYN, BLK, CD22 and CD5 had statistically significant difference (P<0.05). Compared with controls, gene expression levels of CD45, NFAM1, BTK, SYN, and LYN were significantly up-regulated (P<0.05), whereas CD79A, CD21 (P<0.05), FCRL3, CD79B, CD19, CD81, FYN, BLK, CD22, and CD5 (all P<0.01) mRNA expressions were down-regulated in the AMI group. In PBMCs from AMI patients, expressions of the genes including CD45, NFAM1, SYN and LYN were statistically higher (P<0.01) while FCRL3, CD79B, CD19, CD81, FYN, BLK, CD22, and CD5 were significantly lower (P<0.05) than those in PBMCs from the SAP group. Between the SAP and control groups, there were no significant differences in BCR mRNA expressions.

Expression of genes related to activation of T cell independent B cells (B1 cells)

The results showed that mRNA expressions of 7 genes related to B1 cell activation in PBMCs from AMI, SAP patients, and the control group were detected (Figure 12-6-2). In separate comparison with SAP and control patients, CD16, CD32, LILRA1 and TLR9 mRNAs in AMI patients were significantly up-regulated (P<0.05). There was no statistical difference between SAP patients and the controls in T cell independent B cell activation expressions.

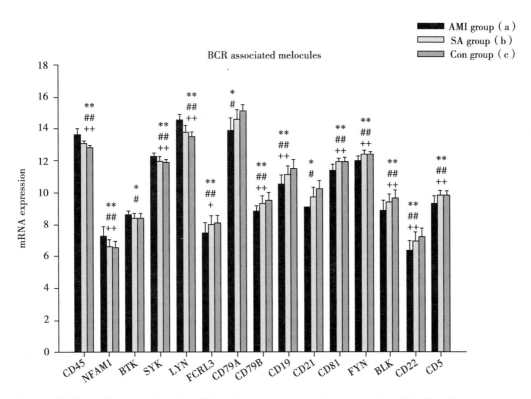

Figure 12-6-1   The significantly differential expression of genes related to B cell receptor in B cell activation in PBMCs from three groups Three groups *P<0.05,**P<0.01. a v c #P<0.05, ##P<0.01.b v c &P<0.05, &&P<0.01. a v b +P<0.05,++P<0.01. (Molecular Medicine Reports, 2016, 13(5):4113-4121)

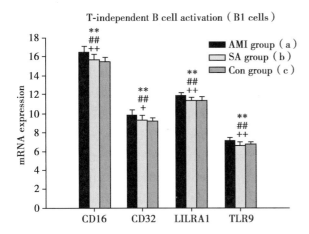

Figure 12-6-2   The significantly differential expression of genes related to T cell independent B cell activation in PBMCs from three groups. Three groups *P<0.05, **P<0.01. a v c #P<0.05, ##P<0.01. b v c.&P<0.05, &&P<0.01. a v b +P<0.05,++P<0.01. (Molecular Medicine Reports, 2016, 13(5):4113-4121)

Expression of genes related to activation of T cell dependent B cells (B2 cells)

Expressions of 20 genes related to B2 cell activation in PBMCs from patients with AMI, SAP and the controls were examined (Figure 12-6-3). In PBMCs from three groups, 11 gene expressions encoding EMR2, CD97, SLAMF1, LY9, CD28, CD43, CD72, ICOSL, PD1,CD40, and CD20 were statistically different (P<0.05). mRNA expressions of EMR2

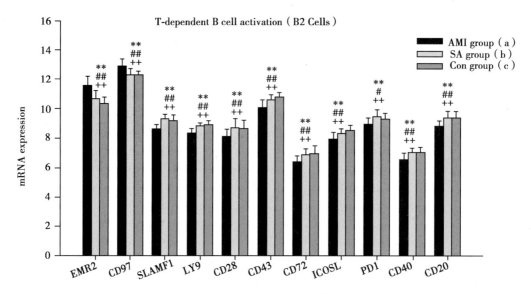

Figure 12-6-3 The significantly differential expression of genes related to T cell dependent B cell activation in PBMCs from three groups. Three groups *P<0.05,**P<0.01. a v c #P<0.05, ##P<0.01. b v c &P<0.05, &&P<0.01. a v b +P<0.05,++P<0.01. (Molecular Medicine Reports, 2016, 13(5):4113-4121)

and CD97 were significantly up-regulated (P<0.01), whereas SLAMF1, LY9, CD28, CD43, CD72, ICOSL, PD1, CD40 and CD20 mRNAs were significantly down-regulated (P<0.05) in AMI patients compared with SAP patients and the controls. There was no significant difference between SAP patients and control group in B2 cell activation mRNA expressions.

Expression of regulators involved in B cell activation

In PBMCs from the AMI and SAP patients and the control group, expressions of 11 genes of regulators involved in B cell activation were examined (Figure 12-6-4), 8 of which were significantly different (P<0.05). In the AMI patients, expressions of the genes including LILRB1, LILRA3 (P <0.05), CR1, LILRB2, LILRB3, and VAV1 (P <0.01) were significantly higher, whereas expressions of CS and IL4I1 were statistically lower (P<0.05) than those from the control group. When compared with the SAP patients, mRNAs of CR1, LILRB2, LILRB3, and VAV1 in AMI patients were significantly up-regulated (P<0.01), while CS1 and IL4I1 mRNAs were significantly down-regulated (P<0.05). There was no significant gene expression difference between SAP patients and the control group in regulators involved in B cell activation.

Expression of genes related to BCR involved in B cell activation

BCR is composed of membrane immunoglobulin (Ig) sheathed by the Igα/Igβ heterodimer. It plays a critical role in mediating B cell development and activation. [13] Ig recognizes the antigens while Igα (CD79A) and Igβ (CD79B) transmits the signals. It was reported that high CD45 expression could reduce the B cell activating factor

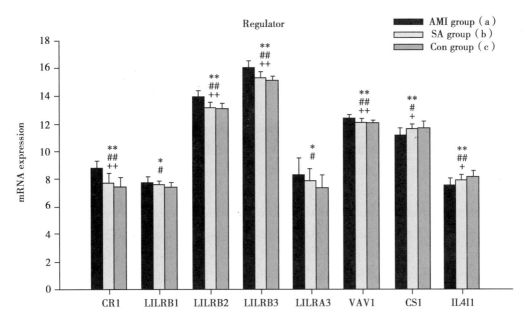

Figure 12-6-4   The significantly differential gene expression of regulators which involved in B cell activation in PBMCs from three groups. Three groups *P<0.05,**P<0.01. a v c #P<0.05, ##P<0.01. b v c &P<0.05, &&P<0.01. a v b +P<0.05,++P<0.01. (Molecular Medicine Reports, 2016, 13(5):4113-4121)

receptor expression and thus inhibit B cell survival. [14,15] *In vivo* studies with mice showed that over expression of NFAM1 could induce severe impairment of early B cell development. [16] Lyn and FCRL3 play both positive and negative roles in B cell activation. [17,18] Genetic ablation of Lyn revealed dominant position in inhibitory roles in B cell signaling. [19] CD19, CD21, CD 81 and FYN are B cell co-receptors and enhance the BCR signal transduction.[20-22] The B cell specific Src-family kinase Blk and CD5, which specifically bind the ligand of B cell surface Ig, are both dispensable for B cell development and activation. [23,24]

In the AMI patients, expressions of CD45, NFAM1 and LYN were significantly higher, while CD79A, CD79B, CD19, CD21, CD81, FYN, BLK and CD5 were oppositely lower than those in control group. The results induced that mRNAs associated with BCR signals were blocked in the AMI patients and might inhibit both B cell activation and development. Comparing SAP patients with the control group, there was no significant difference in BCR antigen recognition mRNAs, demonstrating different BCR antigen recognition activity in AMI and SAP patients.

Expression of genes related to activation of T cell independent B cells (B1 cells)

B1 cells are considered to operate in the innate response to viral and bacterial infections and usually show preferential responses to T cell-independent antigens. [9,11] Among 7 related genes of B1 cells, CD_{16}, CD32, LILRA1 and TLR9 were statistically up-regulated in PBMCs from the AMI patients compared with both SAP and control groups. Studies have shown that Fc gamma receptors CD_{16} and CD32 can influence B cell growth and differentiation.[25,26] Transcripts for LILRA1 were detected in B cells and LILRA1 activated cells by associating with Fc receptor gamma chain.[27,28] Previous studies have demonstrated that human B cells were activated by TLR9 agonist. [29,30] It was therefore suggested that B1 cell activation was enhanced in patients with AMI, indicating that the innate-like response occurred in the AMI patients. However, there was no significant difference in B1 related expression between SAP patients and the control group. All the results suggested the different B1 cell activity in the stages of AMI and SAP.

Expression of genes related to activation of T cell dependent B cells (B2 cells)

B2 cells play a major role in B cell specific humoral immunity.[31] Among the 20 genes examined, expression of EMR2 and CD97 was significantly up-regulated in AMI patients compared with the SAP and control groups. EMR2 and CD97 play a role in the interaction of T cells with B cells.[32] The SLAM family including SLAMF1 and LY9, together with CD28 and CD43, take an essential part in B cell development, maturation, and the control of humoral immune responses.[33-35] The ICOS:ICOSL and PD1:PDL pathways appear to be particularly important for stimulating effector T cell responses and T cell-dependent B cell responses.[36-38] CD40's contact with CD40L expressed on activated T cell surface promotes the activation of B cells.[39] CD20 is a B cell specific integral membrane protein and regulates B cell proliferation.[40] In the present study, SLAMF1, LY9, CD28, CD43, ICOSL, PD1, CD40, and CD20 mRNAs were lower in AMI patients than those in the control group. These results demonstrated that T cell-B ell interaction was weakened in the B2 cell activation in AMI. No significant differences were observed between the SAP patients and the controls, indicating potential insufficiency of humoral responses only in the B2 subset during the stage of AMI.

Gene expression of regulators involved in B cell activation

Among the 11 genes examined, expressions of the genes including CR1, LILRB2, LILRB3, LILRA3 and VAV1 were significantly higher in the AMI patients than those in the SAP and control groups. CR1 is an inhibitor of the BCR mediated B cell activation.[41] LILRB can negatively regulate activation of antigen presenting cells.[42,43] Meanwhile, it has been shown that mice lacking VAV1 had activation defects in B cells.[44] Previous studies showed that CS1 induced proliferation and autocrine cytokine expression on human B lymphocytes.[45] These results demonstrated that B cell activation was inhibited in the patients with AMI. There was no significant gene expression difference between the SAP and control groups in regulators involved in B cell activation.

The statistically significant down-regulation of genes related to BCR, B2 cell subset and regulators in the AMI patients indicated weakened T cell-B cell interaction and blocked B2 cell activation and development. Notably, there was no statistical gene expression difference in all aspects of B cell related genes between the SAP and control groups, demonstrating that the B2 cell subset dysfunction is only observable in the stage of AMI. B2 cell is considered the conventional B lymphocytes, producing and regulating antibody-mediated humoral immunity. Consequently, improving B2 cell mediated humoral immunity may be considered to be a potential target for medical interventions in the patients with AMI.

(published:molecular Medicine Reports 13: 4113-4121, 2016)

References

1. Kyaw T, Tay C, Khan A, Dumouchel V, Cao A, To K, Kehry M, Dunn R, Agrotis A, et al. Conventional B2 B cell depletion ameliorates whereas its aggravates atherosclerosis. J Immunol 185(7):4410-4419, 2010.

2. Clement M, Guedj K, Andreata F, Morvan M, Bey L, Khallou-Laschet J, Gaston AT, Delbosc S,Alsac JM, et al. Control of the T follicular helper-germinal center B-cell axis by CD_8 regulatory T cells limits atherosclerosis and tertiary lymphoid organ development. Circulation 131(6):560-570, 2015.

3. Paigen B, Morrow A, Holmes PA, Mitchell D, Williams RA. Quantitative assessment of atherosclerotic lesions in mice. Atherosclerosis 68(3):231-240,1987.

4. Thorp E, Cui D, Schrijvers DM, Kuriakose G, Tabas I. Mertk receptor mutation reduces efferocytosis efficiency and promotes apoptotic cell accumulation and plaque necrosis in atherosclerotic lesions of apoe-/-mice. Arterioscler Thromb Vasc Biol 28(8):1421-1428, 2008.

5. Tsiantoulas D, Diehl CJ, Witztum JL, Binder CJ.B cells and humoral immunity in atherosclerosis. Circ Res 114(11):1743-1756, 2014.

6. Kyaw T, Tay C, Krishnamurthi S, Kanellakis P, Agrotis A, Tipping P,Bobik A, Toh BH. B1a B lymphocytes are atheroprotective by secreting natural IgM that increases IgM deposits and reduces necrotic cores in atherosclerotic lesions. Circ Res 109:830-840, 2011.

7. Kyaw T, Tay C, Hosseini H, Kanellakis P, Gadowski T, MacKay F, Tipping P, Bobik A, Toh BH. Depletion of B2 but not B1a B cells in BAFF receptor-deficient ApoE mice attenuates atherosclerosis by potently ameliorating arterial inflammation. PLoS One 7(1):e29371, 2012.

8. Ait-Oufella H, Herbin O, Bouaziz JD, Binder CJ, Uyttenhove C, Laurans L, Taleb S, Van Vré E, Esposito B, et al. B cell depletion reduces the development of atherosclerosis in mice. J Exp Med 207:1579-1587, 2010.

9. Janeway CA, Jr, Travers P, Walport M, Shlomchik MJ. Immunobiology. 5th ed. New York: Garland Science; 2001.

10. Sage AP, Mallat Z. Multiple potential roles for B cells in atherosclerosis. Ann Med 46(5):297-303, 2014.

11. Cerutti A, Cols M, Puga I. Marginal zone B cells: virtues of innate-like antibody-producing lymphocytes. Nat Rev Immunol 13:118-132, 2013.

12. Tsiantoulas D, Sage AP, Mallat Z, Binder CJ. Targeting B cells in atherosclerosis: closing the gap from bench to bedside. Arterioscler Thromb Vasc 35(2):296-302, 2015.

13. Kurosaki T. Regulation of BCR signaling. Mol Immunol 48(11):1287-1291, 2011.

14. Huntington ND, Xu Y, Puthalakath H, Light A, Willis SN, Strasser A, Tarlinton DM. CD45 links the B cell receptor with cell survival and is required for the persistence of germinal centers. Nature immunology 7(2):190-198,

2006.

15. Zikherman J, Doan K, Parameswaran R, Raschke W, Weiss A. Quantitative differences in CD45 expression unmask functions for CD45 in B-cell development, tolerance, and survival. Proc Natl Acad Sci U S A 109(1):E3-12, 2012.

16. Ohtsuka M, Arase H, Takeuchi A, Yamasaki S, Shiina R, Suenaga T, Sakurai D, Yokosuka T, Arase N, et al. NFAM1, an immunoreceptor tyrosine-based activation motif-bearing molecule that regulates B cell development and signaling. Proc Natl Acad Sci U S A 101(21):8126-8131, 2004.

17. Scapini P, Pereira S, Zhang H, Lowell CA. Multiple roles of Lyn kinase in myeloid cell signaling and function. Immunol Rev 228(1):23-40, 2009.

18. Li FJ, Schreeder DM, Li R, Wu J, Davis RS. FCRL3 promotes TLR9-induced B-cell activation and suppresses plasma cell differentiation. Eur J Immunol 43(11):2980-92, 2013.

19. Stepanek O, Draber P, Drobek A, Horejsi V, Brdicka T. Nonredundant roles of Src-family kinases and Syk in the initiation of B-cell antigen receptor signaling. J Immunol 190(4):1807-1818, 2013.

20. Barrington RA, Schneider TJ, Pitcher LA, Mempel TR, Ma M, Barteneva NS, Carroll MC. Uncoupling CD21 and CD19 of the B-cell coreceptor. Proc Natl Acad Sci U S A 106(34):14490-14495, 2009.

21. van Zelm MC, Smet J, Adams B, Mascart F, Schandené L, Janssen F, Ferster A, Kuo CC, Levy S, et al.CD81 gene defect in humans disrupts CD19 complex formation and leads to antibody deficiency. J Clin Invest 120(4):1265-1274, 2010.

22. Barua D,Hlavacek WS,Lipniacki T.A computational model for early events in B cell antigen receptor signaling: analysis of the roles of Lyn and Fyn.J Immunol 189(2): 646-658, 2012.

23. Texido G, Su IH, Mecklenbräuker I, Saijo K, Malek SN, Desiderio S, Rajewsky K, Tarakhovsky A. The B-cell-specific Src-family kinase Blk is dispensable for B-cell development and activation. Mol Cell Biol 20(4):1227-1233, 2000.

24. Pospisil R, Silverman GJ, Marti GE, Aruffo A, Bowen MA, Mage RG. CD5 is A potential selecting ligand for B-cell surface immunoglobulin: a possible role in maintenance and selective expansion of normal and malignant B cells. Leuk Lymphoma 36(3-4):353-365, 2000.

25. de Andres B, Mueller AL, Verbeek S, Sandor M, Lynch RG.A regulatory role for Fcgamma receptors CD_{16} and CD32 in the development of murine B cells. Blood 92(8):2823-2829, 1998.

26. Horejs-Hoeck J, Hren A, Mudde GC, Woisetschläger M. Inhibition of immunoglobulin E synthesis through Fc gammaRII (CD32) by a mechanism independent of B-cell receptor co-cross-linking. Immunology 115(3):407-415, 2005.

27. Tedla N, An H, Borges L, Vollmer-Conna U, Bryant K, Geczy C, McNeil HP. Expression of activating and inhibitory leukocyte immunoglobulin-like receptors in rheumatoid synovium: correlations to disease activity. Tissue Antigens 77(4):305-316, 2011.

28. Fanger NA, Borges L, Cosman D. The leukocyte immunoglobulin-like receptors (LIRs): a new family of immune regulators. J Leukoc Biol 66(2):231-236, 1999.

29. Hanten JA, Vasilakos JP, Riter CL, Neys L, Lipson KE, Alkan SS, Birmachu W. Comparison of human B cell activation by TLR7 and TLR9 agonists. BMC Immunol 9: 39, 2008.

30. Yamazaki K, Yamazaki T, Taki S, Miyake K, Hayashi T, Ochs HD, Agematsu K. Potentiation of TLR9 responses for

human naïve B-cell growth through RP105 signaling. Clin Immunol 135(1):125-136, 2010.

31. Hilgendorf I, Theurl I, Gerhardt LM, Robbins CS, Weber GF, Gonen A, Iwamoto Y, Degousee N, Holderried TA,et al. Innate response activator B cells aggravate atherosclerosis by stimulating T helper-1 adaptive immunity. Circulation 129(16):1677-1687, 2014.

32. Kwakkenbos MJ, Pouwels W, Matmati M, Stacey M, Lin HH, Gordon S, van Lier RA, Hamann J. Expression of the largest CD97 and EMR2 isoforms on leukocytes facilitates a specific interaction with chondroitin sulfate on B cells. J Leukoc Biol 77: 112-119, 2005.

33. De Salort J, Sintes J, Llinàs L, Matesanz-Isabel J, Engel P. Expression of SLAM (CD150) cell-surface receptors on human B-cell subsets: from pro-B to plasma cells. Immunol Lett 134(2):129-136, 2011.

34. Reiter R, Pfeffer K. Impaired germinal centre formation and humoral immune response in the absence of CD28 and interleukin-4. Immunology 106(2):222-228, 2002.

35. Galindo-Albarrán AO, Ramírez-Pliego O, Labastida-Conde RG, Melchy-Pérez EI, Liquitaya-Montiel A, Esquivel-Guadarrama FR, Rosas-Salgado G, Rosenstein Y, Santana MA. CD43 signals prepare human T cells to receive cytokine differentiation signals. J Cell Physiol 229(2):172-180, 2014.

36. Chen J, Wang F, Cai Q, Shen S, Chen Y, Hao C, Sun J.A novel anti-human ICOSL monoclonal antibody that enhances IgG production of B cells. Monoclon Antib Immunodiagn Immunother 32(2):125-131, 2013.

37. Greenwald RJ, Freeman GJ, Sharpe AH. The B7 family revisited. Annu Rev Immunol 23:515-548, 2005.

38. Mak TW, Shahinian A, Yoshinaga SK, Wakeham A, Boucher LM, Pintilie M, Duncan G, Gajewska BU, Gronski M, et al. Costimulation through the inducible costimulator ligand is essential for both T helper and B cell functions in T cell-dependent B cell responses. Nat Immunol 4: 765-772, 2003.

39. Nadeau PJ, Roy A, Gervais-St-Amour C, Marcotte MÈ, Dussault N, Néron S. Modulation of CD40-activated B lymphocytes by N-acetylcysteine involves decreased phosphorylation of STAT3. Mol Immunol 49(4):582-592, 2012.

40. Uchida J, Lee Y, Hasegawa M, Liang Y, Bradney A, Oliver JA, Bowen K, Steeber DA, Haas KM, et al. Mouse CD20 expression and function. Int Immunol 16(1):119-129, 2014.

41. Jozsi M, Prechl J, Bajtay Z, Erdei A.Complement receptor type 1 (CD35) mediates inhibitory signals in human B lymphocytes. J Immunol 168: 2782-2728, 2002.

42. Young NT, Waller EC, Patel R, Roghanian A, Austyn JM, Trowsdale J. The inhibitory receptor LILRB1 modulates the differentiation and regulatory potential of human dendritic cells. Blood 111(6):3090-3096, 2008.

43. Howangyin KY, Loustau M, Wu J, Alegre E, Daouya M, Caumartin J, Sousa S, Horuzsko A, Carosella ED, et al. Multimeric structures of HLA-G isoforms function through differential binding to LILRB receptors. Cell Mol Life Sci 69:4041-4049, 2012.

44. Fujikawa K, Miletic AV, Alt FW, Faccio R, Brown T, Hoog J, Fredericks J, Nishi S, Mildiner S, et al. Vav1/2/3-null mice define an essential role for Vav family proteins in lymphocyte development and activation but a differential requirement in MAPK signaling in T and B cells. J Exp Med 198: 1595-1608, 2003.

45. Lee JK, Mathew SO, Vaidya SV, Kumaresan PR, Mathew PA. CS1 (CRACC, CD319) induces proliferation and autocrine cytokine expression on human B lymphocytes. J Immunol 179: 4672-4678, 2007.

7. Comparison of gene expression of Integrin β2 between AMI and SAP patients

The basic pathology of coronary artery disease (CAD) is atherogenesis. It has been shown that atherogenesis is a chronic infectious process involving various kinds of immune cells caused by endothelial cell injuries [1]. The adhesion process which promotes inflammatory reactions is mediated by adhesion molecules among injured intima and activated leukocytes, platelets and endothelial cells [2].

Integrins are heterodimeric cell adhesion molecules involved in immunity, wound healing and hemostasis [3]. There are 24 kinds of integrins formed by non-covalent associations of 18 α and eight β subunits in human body. Integrin β2 is specifically expressed on surface of leukocytes, including αDβ2, αLβ2, αMβ2 and αXβ2. Abnormalities of human integrin β2 gene (ITGB2) expressions could cause changes in adhesion-depended processes, such as chemotaxis, phagocytosis and aggregation.

This study aimed to detect and compare expression intensity of integrin β2 and its related genes among acute myocardial infarction (AMI) patients, stable angina pectoris (SAP) patients and healthy people and analyze gene expression characteristics of integrin β2 on the surface of leukocytes in different phases.

Results

A total of 76 genes associated with integrin β2 were detected. The mRNA expressions in three groups are shown as follows (Figures 12-7-1,2,3,4,5,6,7,8).

α/β subunits

The mRNA expression of α/β subunits associated genes in three groups are shown in Figure 12-7-1. Compared to the control group, the mRNA expressions of genes

Figure 12-7-1 mRNA expression of genes associated with the subunits of β2 integrins. *AMI group vs. control group, P<0.05; **AMI group vs. SAP group, P<0.05; AMI, acute myocardial infarction, SAP: stable angina pectoris. (Acta Medica Mediterranea, 2016, 32: 303)

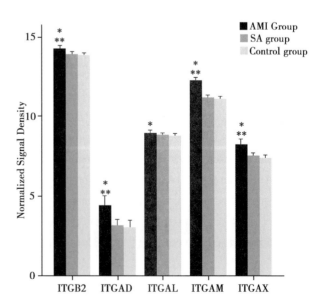

ITGAD, ITGAL, ITGAM, ITGAX and ITGB2 associated with αD, αL, αM, αX and β2 were significantly upregulated (P<0.05); however, there were no significant changes in SAP group (P>0.05). When compared to SAP group, ITGAD, ITGAM, ITGAX and ITGB2 gene expressions were obviously upregulated in AMI group (P<0.05).

Ligands

The mRNA expressions of genes related to ligands of integrin β2 in the three groups are shown in Figure 12-7-2. Compared to the controls, the mRNA expressions of genes related to RAGE, JAM-1, Fibrinogen, ICAM-1, ICAM-3, ICAM-5 and uPAR were significantly upregulated, while genes related to ICAM-2 were obviously down-regulated in the AMI group (P<0.05). In the SAP group, mRNA expressions of genes related to Fibrinogen and ICAM-1 were significantly upregulated, while genes related to RAGE and Laminin 8 were significantly downregulated compared to the controls (P<0.05). When compared to the SAP group, mRNA expressions of genes related to RAGE, JAM-1, ICAM-1, ICAM-3, Laminin 8 and uPAR were obviously upregulated, while genes associated with CAM-2 were significantly downregulated (P<0.05).

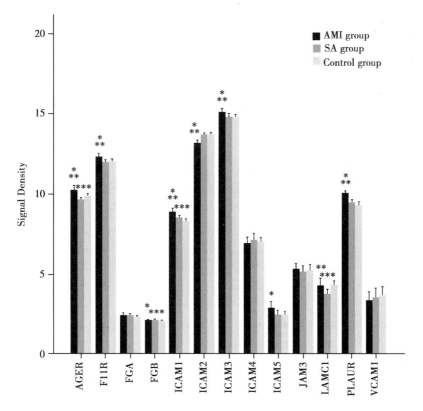

Figure 12-7-2   mRNA expression of genes associated with ligands of β2 integrins. *AMI group vs. control group, P<0.05; **AMI group vs. SAP group, P<0.05; ***SAP group vs. control group, P<0.05; AMI, acute myocardial infarction, SAP: stable angina pectoris. (Acta Medica Mediterranea, 2016, 32: 303)

Chemokines

The mRNA expressions of genes related to chemokines of integrin β2 are shown in Figure 12-7-3. Compared to the control group, the mRNA expressions of genes related to fMLP and RAF were significantly upregulated, while the gene of RANTES was obviously downregulated in the AMI group (P<0.05). However, there were no significant changes in the SAP group compared to control group. When compared to the SAP group, mRNA expression of genes related to RANTES, fMLP and RAF were significantly upregulated in the AMI group (P<0.05).

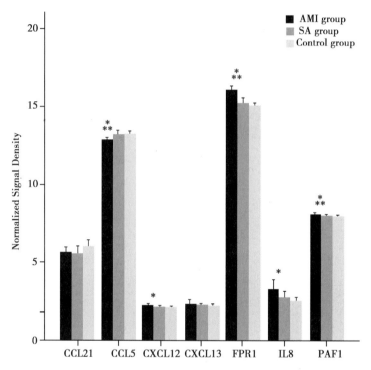

Figure 12-7-3   mRNA expression of genes associated with chemokines. *AMI group vs. control group, P<0.05; **AMI group vs. SAP group, P<0.05; AMI, acute myocardial infarction, SAP: stable angina pectoris. (Acta Medica Mediterranea, 2016, 32: 303)

Inside-out signaling pathway

The mRNA expressions of genes related to Rap-1 in the inside-out signaling pathway of integrin β2 in the three groups are shown in Figure 12-7-4. In the AMI group, the mRNA expressions of genes associated with RIAM, ADAP, SLP-76, PLCγ, RAPL and SPA1 were significantly upregulated, while genes related to Mst1, PLCγ and DalDAG-GEF I were downregulated compared to the control group (P<0.05), while in the SAP group, only mRNA expression of genes related to ADAP was obviously upregulated compared with the controls (P<0.05). When compared with the SAP group, mRNA expression of genes related to RIAM, ADAP, SLP-76, PLCγ, RAPL and SPA1 was

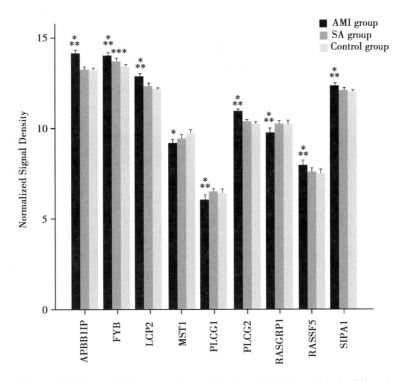

Figure 12-7-4   mRNA expression of Rap1 related signals in inside-out signaling pathway. *AMI group vs. control group, P<0.05; **AMI group vs. SAP group, P<0.05; ***SAP group vs. control group, P<0.05; AMI, acute myocardial infarction, SA: stable angina pectoris. (Acta Medica Mediterranea, 2016, 32: 303)

significantly upregulated, while genes of PLCγ and DalDAG-GEF I were downregulated (P<0.05).

Figure 12-7-5 showed mRNA expressions of genes related to β tails associated proteins and calpain. Compared to the control group, mRNA expressions of genes related to α-actinin, calpain, Dok1, radixin, talin and 14-3-3ζ were significantly upregulated in the AMI group, but genes associated to calpain (CAPN1 and CAPN10), migfilin, talin (TLN2) and vinculin significantly were downregulated (P<0.05). However, mRNA expressions of genes related to β tails associated with proteins and calpain did not change significantly (P>0.05). Compared to SAP group, mRNA expressions of genes related to α-actinin, calpain (CAPN13), Dok1, radixin, talin (TLN1), vinculin and 14-3-3ζ were significantly upregulated (P<0.05), while the gene of CAPN1 was significantly downregulated (P<0.05) in the AMI group.

Proteins in outside-in signaling pathway

The mRNA expressions of genes related to SFK and PKC in the outside-in signaling pathway are shown in Figure 12-7-6. Compared to the control group, genes related to Fgr, Hck, Lyn and PKC (PRKCD, PRKCE and PRKCI) were significantly upregulated,

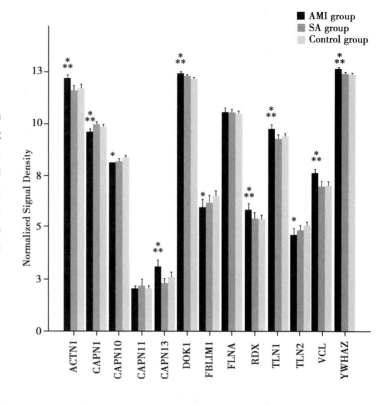

Figure 12-7-5   mRNA expression of other proteins in inside-out signaling pathway. *AMI group vs. control group, P<0.05; **AMI group vs. SAP group, P<0.05; AMI, acute myocardial infarction, SA: stable angina pectoris. (Acta Medica Mediterranea, 2016, 32: 303)

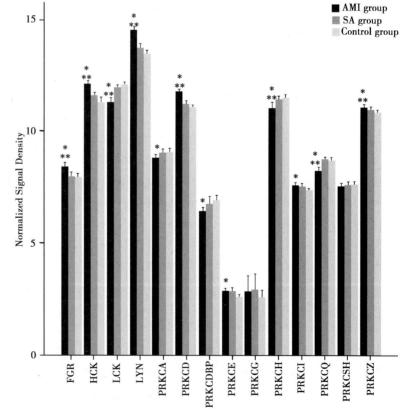

Figure 12-7-6   mRNA expression of SFK and PKC in outside-in signaling pathway. *AMI group vs. control group, P<0.05; **AMI group vs. SAP group, P<0.05; ***SAP group vs. control group, P<0.05; AMI, acute myocardial infarction, SA: stable angina pectoris. (Acta Medica Mediterranea, 2016, 32: 303)

while genes associated with Lck and PKC (PRKCA, PRKCDBP, PRKCH, PRKCQ and RRKCZ) were statistically downregulated in the AMI group (P<0.05). However, mRNA expressions of genes related to Hck, Lyn and PKC (PRKCE and PRKCI) were significantly upregulated in the SAP group when compared to the controls (P<0.05). In the AMI group, mRNA expressions of genes related to Fgr, Hck, Lyn and PKC (PRKCD) were obviously upregulated and genes of Lck and PKC (PRKCH, PRKCQ and RRKCZ) were significantly downregulated when compared to SAP group (P<0.05).

The mRNA expressions of genes associated with SYK in the outside-in signaling pathway are shown in Figure 12-7-7. Compared to the controls, mRNA expressions of genes related to ABL2 and CBL related to c-ab1, gene SYK to Syk and genes VAV1 and VAV3 to Vav1/3 were significantly upregulated in the AMI group (P<0.05). In the SAP group, mRNA expression of gene VAV3 was significantly upregulated while the gene of ABL1 was obviously downregulated compered to the controls (P<0.05). When compared to the SAP group, mRNA expressions of genes ABL2, CBL, PTK2, SYK, VAV1 and VAV3 were significantly upregulated in the AMI group (P<0.05).

mRNA expressions of genes relevant to cytoskeleton remodeling in outside-in

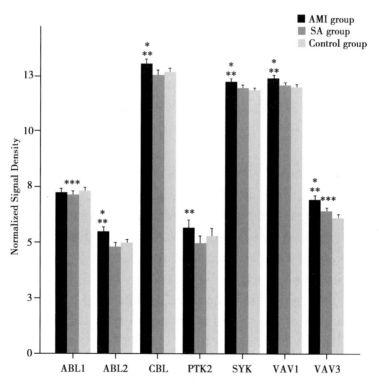

Figure 12-7-7   mRNA expression of genes related to SYK proteins in outside-in signaling pathway *AMI group vs. control group, P<0.05; **AMI group vs. SAP group, P<0.05; ***SAP group vs. control group, P<0.05; AMI, acute myocardial infarction, SA: stable angina pectoris. (Acta Medica Mediterranea, 2016, 32: 303)

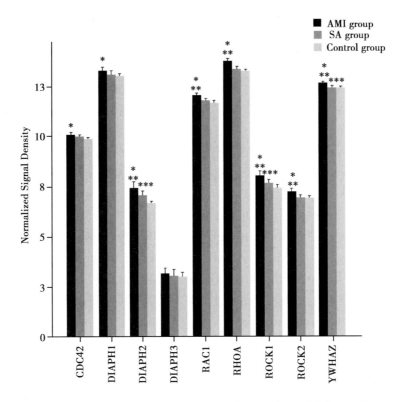

Figure 12-7-8   mRNA expression of proteins which mediate cytoskeleton remodeling in outside-in signaling pathway. *AMI group vs. control group, P<0.05; **AMI group vs. SAP group, P<0.05; ***SAP group vs. control group, P<0.05; AMI, acute myocardial infarction, SA: stable angina pectoris. (Acta Medica Mediterranea, 2016, 32: 303)

signaling pathway were shown in Figure 12-7-8. Compared to the control group, mRNA expressions of genes related to cdc42, Rac, RhoA, ROCK1/2 and genes DIAPH1 and DIAPH2 of mDia were significantly upregulated in the AMI group, while genes DIAPH2 and ROCK1 were upregulated obviously in the SAP group (P<0.05). When compared to the SAP group, the gene of DIAPH2 and genes of Rac, RhoA, ROCK1/2 and 14-3-3ζ were significantly upregulated in the AMI group (P<0.05).

The integrin β2 subunit, which composes of dimers by combining α subunits, is expressed on the surface of leukocytes. β2 subunits were covered by α subunits when inactivated. Its configuration changes and α subunit exposes to its ligands after the β2 subunit is activated. In this study, genes of αDβ2, αLβ2, αMβ2 and αXβ2 were significantly upregulated in the AMI group, while there is no significant change in the SAP group. It is indicated that activation of integrin β2 occurred in acute arterial thrombosis event.

Integrin αLβ2 is expressed on the surface of all kinds of leukocytes and mainly involved in exudation of leukocytes. There are six ligands to integrin αLβ2, including

ICAM-1, ICMA-2, ICAM-3, ICAM-4, ICAM-5 and JAM-1. In the AMI patients, mRNA expression of most genes related to these ligands were obviously upregulated. However, only mRNA expression of ICAM-1 genes was significantly upregulated.

As to integrin αMβ2, it is expressed on bone marrow cells, NK cells and γδ T lymphocytes [4,5]. Ligands to integrin αMβ2 are reported to be CAM-1, Fibrinogen, JAM-3, denatured proteins, inhibitory factor of neutrophil from hookworms, microbial lipopolysaccharide, zymosan, RAGE, uPAR and so on [6-12]. Among them, ligand RAGE is involved in the process of neutrophil adhering to endothelial cells mediated by integrin αMβ2 during acute infections [13]. Reversible compound is formed inside monocytes and on the surface of neutrophils by integrin αMβ2 and GPI anchored uPAR, which binds to its ligand uPA to promote fibrinolysis and clearance of fibrin clot [14-16]. uPAR can also modify the conformation of integrin αMβ2 to regulate the characteristics of ligand binding [14,17-20]. In this study, gene expressions of ICAM-1, Fibrinogen, RAGE and uPAR were significantly upregulated in the AMI patients. However in the SAP group, upregulation of ICAM-1 and downregulation of RAGE was antistatic.

Integrin αXβ2 is mainly expressed on bone marrow cells, dendritic cells, NK cells and activated T and B lymphocytes. Expression of integrin αXβ2 is the symbol of distinguishing mature and immature dendritic cells [21]. The ligands of integrin αXβ2 are almost the same as integrin αMβ2, but integrin αXβ2 is harder to be activated [22]. Gene expressions relative to ligands of integrin αMβ2 were significantly upregulated in the Ami patients, indicating that the ligands were activating integrin αXβ2 the same time of activating integrin αMβ2.

Integrin αDβ2 is highly expressed on foamy macrophages in fatty streak of aorta [23]. The ligands of integrin αDβ2·are only ICAM-2 and VCAM-1 [24,25]. In this study, upregulated ICAM-3 gene expression in AMI patients increased the combination with integrin αDβ2, which activated foamy macrophages.

Inside-out signaling pathway

The Rap1 signaling pathway is the key of the inside-out signaling pathway, which takes part in the process of chemokine activating integrin β2 [26-29]. Rap1 circulates between inactivated GDP combined Rap1 and activated GTP combined Rap1 in the cytoplasm [30]. CalDAG-GEF I and SPA1 play a role in switches between two forms of Rap1 [28,31]. In T lymphocytes, activation of CalDAG-GEF I can upregulate affinity of integrin β2 to its ligands [28], while over expression of SPA1 can cause the opposite results [31]. In AMI patients, gene expression of CalDAG-GEF I was markedly downregulated and SPA1 was upregulated, which inhibited inactivated GDP-Rap1 transformed into activated GTP-Rap1 and reduced affinity of integrin β2 to its ligands.

The characteristic of inside-out signaling pathway is the isolation of tail end inside cells and transmembrane region of α/β subunits, which can be induced by cytoplasm proteins like talin through Rap1 signaling pathway [32-35]. In this study, gene expression of talin was both up and downregulated obviously, which turned out to be imbalanced in AMI patients. Mst has been reported to promote the integrin αLβ2 migrating to the surface of T lymphocytes, but it was downregulated in AMI patients in this study.

The mRNA expression changes of genes related to inside-out signaling pathway indicated that inside-out signaling pathway of integrin β2 in AMI patients was inhibited, however there are no markedly changes in SAP patients.

Outside-in signaling pathway

SFK is demonstrated to play the chief role in outside-in signaling pathway [36] and involvement of Hck, Lyn, c-Yes and Fgr in the pathway is depended on SFK [37-40]. The mRNA expressions of most genes related to SFK were upregulated in AMI patients in this study, indicating that the outside-in signaling pathway was activated.

Besides, phagocytosis is mediated by integrin αMβ2, which is involved in various proteins of cytoskeleton remodeling [41-44]. In AMI patients of this study, the mRNA expressions of genes related to cytoskeleton remodeling were significantly upregulated, suggesting that phagocytosis mediated by integrin αMβ2 was increased, as the same in SAP patients.

In AMI patients, the inside-out signaling pathway of integrin β2 is inhibited while the outside-in signaling pathway is activated, suggesting that activation of integrin β2 in AMI patients might be caused by extracellular factors.

(published: Acta Medica Mediterranea, 2016, 32: 255-264)

References

1. Ikonomidis I, Michalakeas CA, Parissis J, Paraskevaidis I, Ntai K, Papadakis I, Anastasiou-Nana M and Lekakis J. Inflammatory markers in coronary artery disease. Biofactors 2012; 38: 320-328.

2. Hansson GK. Inflammation, atherosclerosis, and coronary artery disease. N Engl J Med 2005; 352: 1685-1695.

3. Hynes RO. Integrins: bidirectional, allosteric signaling machines. Cell 2002; 110: 673-687.

4. Larson RS and Springer TA. Structure and function of leukocyte integrins. Immunol Rev 1990; 114: 181-217.

5. Graff JC and Jutila MA. Differential regulation of CD11b on gammadelta T cells and monocytes in response to unripe apple polyphenols. J Leukoc Biol 2007; 82: 603-607.

6. Plow EF, Haas TA, Zhang L, Loftus J and Smith JW. Ligand binding to integrins. J Biol Chem 2000; 275: 21785-21788.

7. Forsyth CB, Plow EF and Zhang L. Interaction of the fungal pathogen Candida albicans with integrin CD11b/CD18: recognition by the I domain is modulated by the lectin-like domain and the CD18 subunit. J Immunol 1998; 161: 6198-6205.

8. Cywes C, Godenir NL, Hoppe HC, Scholle RR, Steyn LM, Kirsch RE and Ehlers MR. Nonopsonic binding of Mycobacterium tuberculosis to human complement receptor type 3 expressed in Chinese hamster ovary cells.

Infect Immun 1996; 64: 5373-5383.

9. Santoso S, Sachs UJ, Kroll H, Linder M, Ruf A, Preissner KT and Chavakis T. The junctional adhesion molecule 3 (JAM-3) on human platelets is a counterreceptor for the leukocyte integrin Mac-1. J Exp Med 2002; 196: 679-691.

10. Davis GE. The Mac-1 and p150,95 beta 2 integrins bind denatured proteins to mediate leukocyte cell-substrate adhesion. Exp Cell Res 1992; 200: 242-252.

11. Ross GD, Cain JA and Lachmann PJ. Membrane complement receptor type three (CR3) has lectin-like properties analogous to bovine conglutinin as functions as a receptor for zymosan and rabbit erythrocytes as well as a receptor for iC3b. J Immunol 1985; 134: 3307-3315.

12. Rieu P, Ueda T, Haruta I, Sharma CP and Arnaout MA. The A-domain of beta 2 integrin CR3 (CD11b/CD18) is a receptor for the hookworm-derived neutrophil adhesion inhibitor NIF. J Cell Biol 1994; 127: 2081-2091.

13. Frommhold D, Kamphues A, Hepper I, Pruenster M, Lukic IK, Socher I, Zablotskaya V, Buschmann K, Lange-Sperandio B, Schymeinsky J, Ryschich E, Poeschl J, Kupatt C, Nawroth PP, Moser M, Walzog B, Bierhaus A and Sperandio M. RAGE and ICAM-1 cooperate in mediating leukocyte recruitment during acute inflammation *in vivo*. Blood 2010; 116: 841-849.

14. Simon DI, Rao NK, Xu H, Wei Y, Majdic O, Ronne E, Kobzik L and Chapman HA. Mac-1 (CD11b/CD18) and the urokinase receptor (CD87) form a functional unit on monocytic cells. Blood 1996; 88: 3185-3194.

15. Pluskota E, Soloviev DA and Plow EF. Convergence of the adhesive and fibrinolytic systems: recognition of urokinase by integrin alpha Mbeta 2 as well as by the urokinase receptor regulates cell adhesion and migration. Blood 2003; 101: 1582-1590.

16. Pluskota E, Soloviev DA, Bdeir K, Cines DB and Plow EF. Integrin alphaMbeta2 orchestrates and accelerates plasminogen activation and fibrinolysis by neutrophils. J Biol Chem 2004; 279: 18063-18072.

17. Simon DI, Wei Y, Zhang L, Rao NK, Xu H, Chen Z, Liu Q, Rosenberg S and Chapman HA. Identification of a urokinase receptor-integrin interaction site. Promiscuous regulator of integrin function. J Biol Chem 2000; 275: 10228-10234.

18. Tang ML, Kong LS, Law SK and Tan SM. Down-regulation of integrin alpha M beta 2 ligand-binding function by the urokinase-type plasminogen activator receptor. Biochem Biophys Res Commun 2006; 348: 1184-1193.

19. Zhang H, Colman RW and Sheng N. Regulation of CD11b/CD18 (Mac-1) adhesion to fibrinogen by urokinase receptor (uPAR). Inflamm Res 2003; 52: 86-93.

20. Tang ML, Vararattanavech A and Tan SM. Urokinase-type plasminogen activator receptor induces conformational changes in the integrin alphaMbeta2 headpiece and reorientation of its transmembrane domains. J Biol Chem 2008; 283: 25392-25403.

21. O'Doherty U, Peng M, Gezelter S, Swiggard WJ, Betjes M, Bhardwaj N and Steinman RM. Human blood contains two subsets of dendritic cells, one immunologically mature and the other immature. Immunology 1994; 82: 487-493.

22. Zang Q and Springer TA. Amino acid residues in the PSI domain and cysteine-rich repeats of the integrin beta2 subunit that restrain activation of the integrin alpha(X)beta(2). J Biol Chem 2001; 276: 6922-6929.

23. Van der Vieren M, Le Trong H, Wood CL, Moore PF, St John T, Staunton DE and Gallatin WM. A novel leukointegrin, alpha d beta 2, binds preferentially to ICAM-3. Immunity 1995; 3: 683-690.

24. Wu H, Rodgers JR, Perrard XY, Perrard JL, Prince JE, Abe Y, Davis BK, Dietsch G, Smith CW and Ballantyne CM. Deficiency of CD11b or CD11d results in reduced staphylococcal enterotoxin-induced T cell response and T cell phenotypic changes. J Immunol 2004; 173: 297-306.

25. Grayson MH, Van der Vieren M, Sterbinsky SA, Michael Gallatin W, Hoffman PA, Staunton DE and Bochner BS. alphadbeta2 integrin is expressed on human eosinophils and functions as an alternative ligand for vascular cell adhesion molecule 1 (VCAM-1). J Exp Med 1998; 188: 2187-2191.

26. Katagiri K, Hattori M, Minato N, Irie S, Takatsu K and Kinashi T. Rap1 is a potent activation signal for leukocyte function-associated antigen 1 distinct from protein kinase C and phosphatidylinositol-3-OH kinase. Mol Cell Biol 2000; 20: 1956-1969.

27. Tohyama Y, Katagiri K, Pardi R, Lu C, Springer TA and Kinashi T. The critical cytoplasmic regions of the alphaL/beta2 integrin in Rap1-induced adhesion and migration. Mol Biol Cell 2003; 14: 2570-2582.

28. Ghandour H, Cullere X, Alvarez A, Luscinskas FW and Mayadas TN. Essential role for Rap1 GTPase and its guanine exchange factor CalDAG-GEFI in LFA-1 but not VLA-4 integrin mediated human T-cell adhesion. Blood 2007; 110: 3682-3690.

29. Ebisuno Y, Katagiri K, Katakai T, Ueda Y, Nemoto T, Inada H, Nabekura J, Okada T, Kannagi R, Tanaka T, Miyasaka M, Hogg N and Kinashi T. Rap1 controls lymphocyte adhesion cascade and interstitial migration within lymph nodes in RAPL-dependent and-independent manners. Blood 2010; 115: 804-814.

30. Rousseau-Merck MF, Pizon V, Tavitian A and Berger R. Chromosome mapping of the human RAS-related RAP1A, RAP1B, and RAP2 genes to chromosomes 1p12—p13, 12q14, and 13q34, respectively. Cytogenet Cell Genet 1990; 53: 2-4.

31. Shimonaka M, Katagiri K, Nakayama T, Fujita N, Tsuruo T, Yoshie O and Kinashi T. Rap1 translates chemokine signals to integrin activation, cell polarization, and motility across vascular endothelium under flow. J Cell Biol 2003; 161: 417-427.

32. Garcia-Alvarez B, de Pereda JM, Calderwood DA, Ulmer TS, Critchley D, Campbell ID, Ginsberg MH and Liddington RC. Structural determinants of integrin recognition by talin. Mol Cell 2003; 11: 49-58.

33. Wegener KL, Partridge AW, Han J, Pickford AR, Liddington RC, Ginsberg MH and Campbell ID. Structural basis of integrin activation by talin. Cell 2007; 128: 171-182.

34. Anthis NJ, Wegener KL, Ye F, Kim C, Goult BT, Lowe ED, Vakonakis I, Bate N, Critchley DR, Ginsberg MH and Campbell ID. The structure of an integrin/talin complex reveals the basis of inside-out signal transduction. Embo j 2009; 28: 3623-3632.

35. Shattil SJ, Kim C and Ginsberg MH. The final steps of integrin activation: the end game. Nat Rev Mol Cell Biol 2010; 11: 288-300.

36. Sarantos MR, Zhang H, Schaff UY, Dixit N, Hayenga HN, Lowell CA and Simon SI. Transmigration of neutrophils across inflamed endothelium is signaled through LFA-1 and Src family kinase. J Immunol 2008; 181: 8660-8669.

37. Xue ZH, Zhao CQ, Chua GL, Tan SW, Tang XY, Wong SC and Tan SM. Integrin alphaMbeta2 clustering triggers phosphorylation and activation of protein kinase C delta that regulates transcription factor Foxp1 expression in monocytes. J Immunol 2010; 184: 3697-3709.

38. Giagulli C, Ottoboni L, Caveggion E, Rossi B, Lowell C, Constantin G, Laudanna C and Berton G. The Src family

kinases Hck and Fgr are dispensable for inside-out, chemoattractant-induced signaling regulating beta 2 integrin affinity and valency in neutrophils, but are required for beta 2 integrin-mediated outside-in signaling involved in sustained adhesion. J Immunol 2006; 177: 604-611.

39. Lowell CA, Fumagalli L and Berton G. Deficiency of Src family kinases p59/61hck and p58c-fgr results in defective adhesion-dependent neutrophil functions. J Cell Biol 1996; 133: 895-910.

40. Totani L, Piccoli A, Manarini S, Federico L, Pecce R, Martelli N, Cerletti C, Piccardoni P, Lowell CA, Smyth SS, Berton G and Evangelista V. Src-family kinases mediate an outside-in signal necessary for beta2 integrins to achieve full activation and sustain firm adhesion of polymorphonuclear leucocytes tethered on E-selectin. Biochem J 2006; 396: 89-98.

41. Caron E and Hall A. Identification of two distinct mechanisms of phagocytosis controlled by different Rho GTPases. Science 1998; 282: 1717-1721.

42. Wheeler AP and Ridley AJ. Why three Rho proteins? RhoA, RhoB, RhoC, and cell motility. Exp Cell Res 2004; 301: 43-49.

43. Watanabe N, Kato T, Fujita A, Ishizaki T and Narumiya S. Cooperation between mDia1 and ROCK in Rho-induced actin reorganization. Nat Cell Biol 1999; 1: 136-143.

44. Kovar DR, Harris ES, Mahaffy R, Higgs HN and Pollard TD. Control of the assembly of ATP-and ADP-actin by formins and profilin. Cell 2006; 124: 423-435.

Chapter 13

The impaired innate and adaptive immunity in patients with coronary artery diseases

Cardiovascular diseases (CADs), with high morbidity and mortality worldwide, are caused mainly by atherosclerosis. In particular, acute myocardial infarction (AMI) represents life-threatening conditions during the history of CAD [1,2]. Nowadays we are still unable to effectively predict and prevent AMI occurrence. The pathologic mechanism responsible for the majority of AMI is the rupture of stable atherosclerotic plaque and then with thrombosis [3]. Obviously, there must be a trigger to induce the sudden rupture. Infection seems to be undoubtedly linked to vulnerable atherosclerotic lesions; however, its role cannot be easily documented [4-6]. Various exogenous microorganisms' infections, including Chlamydia pneumoniae, *Helicobacter pylori*, Cytomegalovirus and *Bacteroides gingivalis* are accepted as the new risk factors of CAD [7,8].

Our recent study demonstrated the decreased T cell immunity function in AMI patients [9,10]. T cell is a key component of adaptive immune system, which eliminates the pathogenic microorganisms and malignant cells. The significant decline of T cell function suggested that the pathogenesis of acute thrombosis in AMI patients may be associated with the depletion of immune cells. However, little is known about the nature of immune response in different stages of CAD [11,12]. In resent study, we designed this *in vitro* study to investigate both innate and adaptive immunity in patients with AMI and stable angina pectoris (SAP). Human microarray analysis was used to systematically measure the mRNA expression of the complement component, the markers of immune cells in peripheral blood mononuclear cells (PBMCs) from AMI, SAP and controls. Moreover, the quantity of immune cells, related cytokines and immunoglobulin levels were also measured.

Patients' Information

The study recruited 210 patients with AMI, 210 with SAP, and 250 clinical controls. Human microarray analysis was performed for 20 randomly chosen subjects per group. The sample sizes and the number of subjects per group were based on an assumed within-group variance of 0.50 and the targeted nominal power of 0.95 [13]. Table13-1-1 shows the baseline demographic data. All the patients were enrolled between Mar 2013 and Feb 2015 from our Coronary Care Unit and Cardiovascular Department. The AMI patients were admitted no more than 12 hours from the onset of symptoms to our Coronary Care Unit including 180 males and 30 females, with an average age of 59±11 (mean±s.d.) years. The SAP group has 210 patients (176 male, 34 female, age 64±11). 250 in patients (207 male, 43 female, age 61±9) were enrolled as the control group during the same period. Histories, physical examination, ECG, chest radiography and routine chemical analyses showed the controls had no evidence of coronary heart diseases.

All AMI patients were diagnosed on the basis of the following criteria [14]: Detection of a rise of cardiac biomarker values [preferably cardiac troponin (cTn)] with at least one value above the 99th percentile upper reference limit (URL) and with at least one of the following: 1) Symptoms of ischemia. 2) New or presumed new significant ST-segment-T wave (ST-T) changes or new left bundle branch block (LBBB). 3) Development of pathological Q waves in ECG. 4) Imaging evidence of new loss of viable myocardium or new regional wall motion abnormality. 5) Identification of an intracoronary thrombus by angiography.

All SAP patients had exclusively effort-related angina with a positive exercise stress test and at least one coronary stenosis was detected at angiography (>70% reduction of lumen diameter).

There were no significant differences among the three groups in age, sex, body mass index (BMI), ethnicity, smoking status, systolic blood pressure (SBP), diastolic blood pressure (DBP), low-density lipoprotein cholesterol (LDL-C), triglycerides, high-density lipoprotein cholesterol (HDL-C) or fasting plasma glucose (FBG) (Table 13-1-1).

Table13-1-1　Baseline demographic data in three groups ($\bar{x}$±s.d.)

Index	AMI (a) (N=210)	SAP(b) (N=210)	Con(c) (N=250)	P(all)	P(a v b)
Age	58.5±10.7	63.6±11.1	60.9±9.4	0.141	0.211
Sex(M/F)	180/30	176/34	207/43	0.694	0.773
BMI(kg/m^2)	24.6±2.9	22.5±2.2	22.7±1.9	0.112	0.76
Ethnicity, Han	210	210	250	1	1
Tobacco smoking (num/d)	13.6±10.1	14.4.±8.4	11.2±6.1	0.24	0.648
SBP (mmHg)	130.1±11.3	123.7±10.1	124.8±7.8	0.145	0.701
DBP (mmHg)	67.7±8.8	72.0±8.8	77.6±3.6	0.126	0.24
LDL-C (mmol/L)	2.8±1.2	2.4±1.8	2.7±1.5	0.44	0.676
Triglycerides (mmol/L)	1.5±1.8	1.7±1.0	1.8±0.7	0.51	0.12
HDL-C (mmol/L)	0.7±0.9	0.8±0.7	0.9±0.2	0.11	0.303
FBG (mmol/L)	5.3±0.4	5.1±0.7	5.0±0.2	0.24	0.834

Footnotes: BMI= body mass index; SBP=systolic blood pressure; DBP =diastolic blood pressure; LDL-C=low-density lipoprotein cholesterol; HDL-C: high-density lipoprotein cholesterol; FBG: Fasting Plasma Glucose

The exclusion criteria for the three groups were as follows: venous thrombosis, history of severe renal or hepatic diseases, hematological disorders, acute or chronic inflammatory diseases and malignancy.

The study protocol was approved by the ethics committee of Tongji University and informed consent form was obtained.

Gene Expression Chips

Agilent G4112F Whole Human Genome Oligo Microarrays purchased from Agilent (USA) were used in the chip analysis. A microarray is composed of more than 41,000 genes or transcripts, including targeted 19,596 entrez gene RNAs. Sequence information used in the microarrays was derived from the latest databases of RefSeq, Goldenpath, Ensembl and Unigene [15]. More than 70% of the gene functions in the microarray are already known. All 20 randomly selected patients for each group were subjected to the chip analysis.

Total RNA Isolation

Ten milliliter of peripheral blood samples from median cubital vein were drawn from all the patients immediately after admission. Four milliliter blood was kept in PAXgene tube for total RNA isolation and the rest six milliliter was for laboratory assays. Leucocytes were obtained through density gradient centrifugation with Ficoll solution and the remaining red blood cells were destroyed by erythrocyte lysis buffer (Qiagen, Hilden, Germany). Following the manufacturer's instructions, total RNA was extracted and purified using PAXgene TM Blood RNA kit (Cat#762174, QIAGEN, GmBH, Germany). It was further checked for a RIN number to inspect RNA integration by an Agilent Bioanalyzer 2100 (Agilent technologies, Santa Clara, CA, US). The sample was considered qualified when both 2100 RIN and 28S/18S were larger than or equal to 0.7.

RNA Amplification and Labeling

Total RNA was amplified and labeled by Low Input Quick Amp Labeling Kit, One-Color (Cat#5190-2305, Agilent technologies, Santa Clara, CA, US), following the manufacturer's instructions. Labeled cRNA was purified by RNeasy mini kit (Cat#74106, QIAGEN, GmBH, Germany).

Microarray Hybridization

Each slide was hybridized with 1.65ìg Cy3-labeled cRNA using Gene Expression Hybridization Kit (Cat#5188-5242, Agilent technologies, Santa Clara, CA, US) in Hybridization Oven (Cat#G2545A, Agilent technologies, Santa Clara, CA, US), following the manufacturer's instructions. After 17 hours of hybridization, slides were washed in staining dishes (Cat#121, Thermo Shandon, Waltham, MA, US) with Gene Expression

Wash Buffer Kit(Cat#5188-5327, Agilent technologies, Santa Clara, CA, US),according to the manufacturer's operation manual.

Chip Scan and Data Acquisition

Slides were scanned using Agilent Microarray Scanner (Cat#G2565CA, Agilent technologies, Santa Clara, CA, US) with default settings. Dye channel: Green, Scan resolution=3ìm, 20bit. Data were extracted with Feature Extraction software 10.7 (Agilent technologies, Santa Clara, CA, US). Raw data were normalized using Quantile algorithm, Gene Spring Software 11.0 (Agilent technologies, Santa Clara, CA, US).

RT-PCR

The spots in the microarray were randomly selected and their expressions were confirmed by RT-PCR. Among all the genes with different expressions, three genes were randomly selected and subjected to RT-PCR, along with the house keeping genes (GAPDH). The relative expressions were indicated as the expression of the target genes normalized to the expression of GAPDH (2-ÄÄCt). The melting curve and the 2-ÄÄCt-method were used to detect the differences in the expressions among the three groups. The results from RT-PCR were consistent with the microarray analysis.

Laboratory assays

Two milliliter blood sample was anticoagulated with EDTA-K3 for the counting of $CD_{16}CD_{56}$ natural killer cells, T lymphocyte subsets and CD_{19} B cells, and the rest four milliliter was separated by centrifugation within 1 hour for the examination of serum immunoglobulin and cytokines. All tests were finished within two weeks.

CH50 was detected with liposome immune assay (Beckmann DxC-800 fully automatic biochemical analyzer, USA; Reagents: Wako Pure Chemical Industries, Ltd., Japan). C3 and C4 were detected with immunone-phelometry (BNII system, Siemens AG, Germany; Reagents: Siemens Healthcare Diagnostics Products GmbH,Germany).

Cytokines, including IL-2, IL-4, IL-6 and IFN-γ, were measured by double antibody sandwich ELISA assay (Microplate reader Model 2010, Anthos, Austria; Reagents: Dili biotech, Shanghai). Serum levels of IgA, IgM and IgG were calculated by the immunonephelometric technique using the automated IMMAGE 800 immunochemistry system (Beckman Coulter, Brea, CA, USA), and expressed as g/L.

Leukocyte subpopulations were measured by flow cytometry (BEPICS XL-4, BECKMAN-COULTER). Monoclonal antibodies against CD_3, CD_4, CD_8, CD_{16}, CD_{56} and CD_{19} were purchased from BD Biosciences. The antibodies were marked with one of three fluorochromes: fluorescein isothiocyanate (FITC), phycoerythrin (PE) and phycoerythrin-cyanin 5.1 (PC5). The cells were identified by combinations as follows: CD_3 (FITC)/CD_{16} (PE)/CD_{56} (PC5) (NK cells), CD_3 (FITC)/CD_4 (PE)/CD_8 (PC5) (CD_4 and CD_8

cells), and CD_{19} (PE) (B cells). In brief, 100 μL of EDTA treated blood was added to each tube and the control tube was also included. 20 μL of mouse IgG1-FITC, IgG1-PE or IgG1-PC5 was then added, followed by addition of corresponding fluorescence antibodies. Following vortexing, incubation was done in dark for 30 min at room temperature. 500 μL of hemolysin (BECKMAN-COULTER) was then added, followed by incubation at 37°C for 30 min. Following washing, 500 μL of sheath fluid was added to each tube, followed by flow cytometry (EPICS XL-4, BECKMAN-COULTER). The PMT voltage, fluorescence compensation and sensitivity of standard fluorescent microspheres (EPICS XL-4, BECKMAN-COULTER) were used to adjust the flow cytometer and a total of 10,000 cells were counted for each tube. The corresponding cell population in the scatter plot of isotype controls was used to set the gate, and the proportion of positive cells was determined in each quadrant (%). SYSTEM-Ⅱ was used to process the data obtained after flow cytometry.

Statistical Analysis

Descriptive statistics were expressed as mean±s.d. Differences between groups were examined by one-way analysis of variance (ANOVA). After ANOVA the test of all pairwise group mean comparison was performed using the Tukey's method. Density curves for CH50, C3, C4, $CD_{16}CD_{56}$, CD_3, CD_4, CD_8 and CD_{19} cells were delineated using R software. Data were analyzed using SPSS 17.0, and p-values <0.05 were considered statistically significant.

Results

Gene expression and serum level of the complement

The results showed mRNA expressions of early and late complement components including C1qá, C1qâ, C1qγ, C1r, C1s, C2, C3, C4b, C5a, C6, C7, C8á, C8â, C8γ and C9 were examined in PBMCs from the three groups of patients (Figure 13-1-1A). In AMI group gene expressions of C1qá (P<0.05), C1qâ, C1qγ, C1r and C5a (all P<0.01) were significantly up-regulated, whereas expressions of C7, C8â and C9 were significantly down-regulated when compared with SAP patients and controls respectively (P<0.05). C1s expression in AMI patients was lower than the controls (P<0.05). The serum CH50, C3 and C4 levels were significantly increased in AMI and SAP patients when compared with controls (P<0.01). CH50 was higher in AMI patients than in SAP patients (P<0.01). There was no significant difference between AMI and SAP patients in C3 and C4 levels. The density curves of CH50, C3 and C4 were shown in Figure 13-1-1B, C, D separately.

Gene expression and counting of NK cells

The results showed 12 gene expressions of NK cell biomarkers [16], including CD16, CD56, five inhibitory receptors, CD94, NKG2A, CD158(KIR2DL), CD161 (KLRB1), CD328 (Siglect-7) and five activating NK cell receptors, including CD335 (Nkp46), CD337

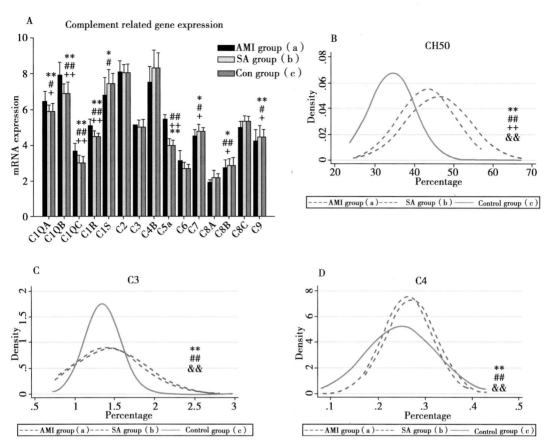

Figure 13-1-1   From three groups in PBMCs, (A) mRNA expression of early and late components complement. (B) Serum CH50 level. (C) Serum C3 level. (D) Serum C4 level. Three groups: *P<0.05; **P<0.01.a v c: #P<0.05; ##P<0.01. a v b: +P<0.05; ++P<0.01. b v c &P<0.05; &&P<0.01. (International Journal Of Medical Sciences, 2017,14(2):181-190)

(Nkp30), CD48 (2B4), CD314 (NKG2D) and CD319 (CRACC) in PBMCs from the three groups (Figure 13-1-2 A). In the AMI group mRNA expressions of the genes encoding CD94, NKG2A, CD158, CD161, CD337, CD314 and CD319 were significantly lower (P<0.05) than in SAP patients and the controls. There was no statistical difference in NK cell biomarker expressions between SAP and the controls. Density curves for the NK cell proportion in PBMCs from three groups were delineated (Figure 13-1-2B). The two density curves of cell proportion from AMI and SAP patients in PBMCs were substantially left shift when compared with the controls. The number of NK cells was significantly decreased in both AMI and SAP patients (P<0.01). However, there was no significant difference between the AMI and SAP patients in the quantity of NK cells.

Gene expression, subsets counting and related cytokines of T cells

Expressions of 8 genes related to T cell receptor (TCR) antigen recognition, 16

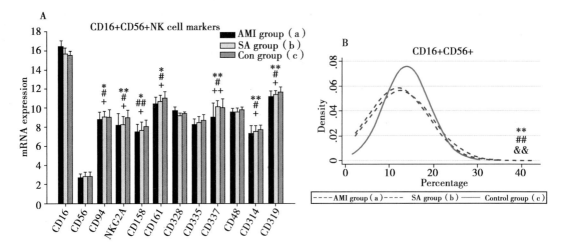

Figure 13-1-2   From three groups in PBMCs, (A) mRNA expression of intracellular and extracellular markersof $CD_{16}CD_{56}$cells. (B) The comparison of $CD_{16}CD_{56}$ cells counting. Three groups: *P<0.05; **P<0.01.a v c: #P<0.05; ##P<0.01. a v b: +P<0.05; ++P<0.01. b v c: &P<0.05; &&P<0.01. (International Journal Of Medical Sciences, 2017,14(2):181-190)

genes associated with CD_4T cells and 15 genes with CD_8 T cells were detected among three groups (Figure 13-1-3A, C, E). 16 genes in AMI patients encoding TCRA, TCRB, TCRG, TCRZ, CD3D, CD3E, CD3G, CD195(CCR5), IL-10, GATA3, CD278(ICOS), CD8A, CD8B, CD28, GZMM and CASP10 were significantly down-regulated when compared with the SAP patients and controls respectively (P<0.05). TCRIM, CD294 (CRTH2) and GZMK expressions in AMI group were significantly lower than those in SAP group (P<0.05). Comparing with controls, gene expressions of CD_4, IL4 and TNFA in AMI group were significantly down-regulated (P<0.05), while IL-2 and CD366 (Tim-3) mRNA expressions were up-regulated (P<0.05). Between the SAP and control groups, there was no statistical difference in TCR, CD_4 and CD_8T cell markers related mRNA expression.

Results from the proportions of cytological T lymphocyte subsets in PBMCs among three groups showed that the levels of CD_3 and CD_8T cells in AMI and SAP group were decreased significantly (P< 0.05), while CD_4T cells increased (P<0.01) when compared with the control group (Figure 13-1-3B,D,F, Table13-1-2). The cytokines IL-2, IL-4, IL-6 and IFN were significantly increased in the AMI and SAP patients when compared with the controls (P<0.01). However, there was no significant difference between the AMI and SAP patients in IL-2, IFN, CD3 T cell and CD_8T cell quantity (Table 13-1-2). The counting of CD_4 T cells, IL-4 and IL-6 were higher in the AMI patients than in the SAP patients (P<0.01).

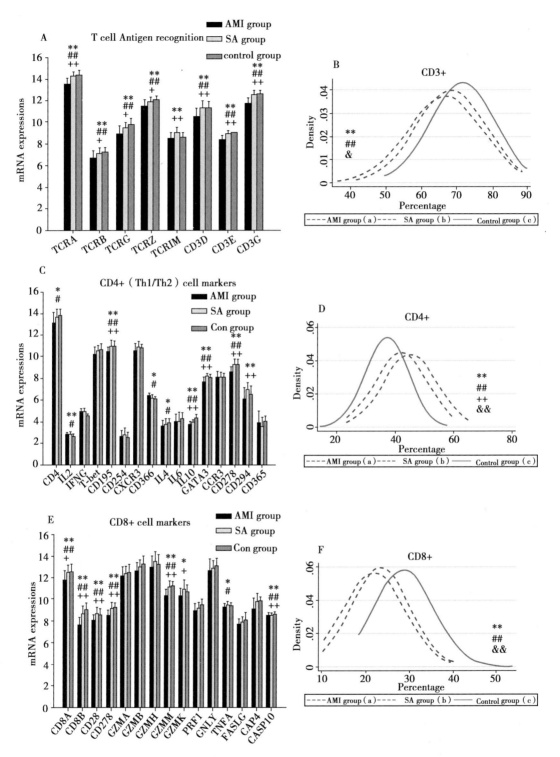

Figure 13-1-3   From three groups in PBMCs, (A) Expression of genes related to T cell antigen recognition. (B) CD₃ counting. (C) Expression of genes related to CD₄. (D) CD₄ counting. (E) Genes related to CD₈. (F) CD₈ counting. Three groups: *P<0.05; **P<0.01.a v c: #P<0.05; ##P<0.01. a v b: +P<0.05; ++P<0.01. b v c: &P<0.05; &&P<0.01. (International Journal Of Medical Sciences, 2017,14(2):181-190)

Table 13-1-2   Values of T cell immunity among three groups ($\bar{x}\pm$s.d.)

Index	AMI (a) (N=210)	SAP (b) (N=210)	Con(c) (N=250)	P(all)	P (a/c)	P(b/c)	P(a/b)
CD$_3$ (%)	66.7±10.7	68.4±10.0	71.5±9.2	0.00	0.00	0.002	0.275
CD$_4$ (%)	42.1±8.9	45.1.±9.2	37.0±9.1	0.00	0.00	0.00	0.003
CD$_8$ (%)	21.8±7.1	23.3±6.7	28.6±6.9	0.00	0.00	0.00	0.068
IL-2 (pg/ml)	34.2±18.5	33.5±14.5	9.9±2.3	0.00	0.00	0.00	0.96
IL-4(pg/ml)	35.7±15.7	28.22±10.9	4.8±2.3	0.00	0.00	0.00	0.00
IL-6 (pg/ml)	29.9±16.2	24.6±14.4	3.0±1.4	0.00	0.00	0.00	0.001
IFN (pg/ml)	40.8±21.4	33.0±22.1	16.7±6.3	0.00	0.00	0.00	0.72

Gene expression, counting and serum immunoglobulin level of B cells

The results showed that expressions of 15 genes related to B cell biomarkers in patients with AMI, SAP and the controls (Figure 13-1-4A), including CD5, CD19, CD20, CD21 (CR1), CD22, CD23, CD40, CD79a, CD79b, CD80(B7-1), CD86(B7-2), CD138, CD154 (IgM), CD268 (BAFFR) and CD279 (PD-1). In the PBMCs from the three groups, expressions of 8 genes encoding CD5, CD19, CD20, CD22, CD40, CD79b, CD268 and CD279 in the AMI group were significantly lower (P<0.05) than those from the SAP and control groups. Compared with controls, gene expressions of CD21, CD23 and CD79a were significantly down-regulated (P<0.05) in AMI patients. Between the SAP and control groups, there were no significant differences in B cell marker expressions. When

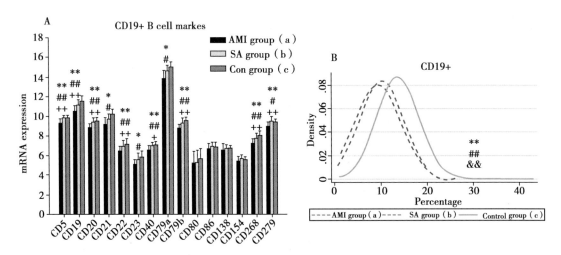

Figure. 13-1-4   From three groups in PBMCs, (A) mRNA expression of intracellular and extracellular markers of CD$_{19}$ cell. (B) The comparison of CD$_{19}$ cells counting. Three groups: *P<0.05; **P<0.01. a v c: #P<0.05; ##P<0.01. a v b: +P<0.05; ++P<0.01. b v c: &P<0.05; &&P<0.01. (International Journal Of Medical Sciences, 2017,14(2):181-190)

compared with controls, B cell counting, IgG and IgM in PBMCs were significantly down-regulated (P<0.01), while IgA was significantly increased (P<0.05) in both AMI and SAP groups (Figure 13-1-4B, Table 13-1-3).

Table13-1-3   Values of B cell immunity among three groups ($\bar{x}$±s.d.)

Index	AMI(a) (N=210)	SAP (b) (N=210)	Con (c) (N=250)	P (all)	P (a/c)	P (b/c)	P (a/b)
CD_{19}(%)	9.4±5.0	10.3±4.7	13.7±4.6	0.00	0.00	0.00	0.212
IgA (g/L)	2.3±1.0	2.2±0.8	1.9±0.7	0.00	0.001	0.014	0.487
IgM (g/L)	0.8±0.42	0.8±0.35	1.2±0.41	0.00	0.00	0.00	0.572
IgG (g/L)	10.8±2.6	11.2±2.2	12.0±2.3	0.00	0.00	0.001	0.242

In our current study, the significantly up-regulated mRNAs expressions of early complement components, C1qá, C1qâ, C1q γ, C1r and C5a demonstrated that the classical pathways were activated in AMI patients. The initiation of classical pathway eventually results in the terminal access to form C5b-9 complex, which makes a transmembrane pore in the target cells' membrane to lysis [17]. C5b initiates the formation of MAC, which consists of C5b, C6, C7, C8, and multiple molecules of C9. In our study the significantly lower levels of C7, C8â and C9 mRNAs in AMI patients suggested the obstacle of MAC formation. In AMI and SAP patients, the serum levels of C3, C4 and CH50, which reflected the activities of C1-C9 via classic pathway, were all elevated. Gene and cytology levels of the complement in both AMI and SAP patients were activated and the results were consistent with previous studies [18-20]. Though the complement was activated in AMI and SAP stages, based on the genomics results of complement cascade reaction imbalance, cytolytic effect of the complement only decreased in AMI patients.

The NK cells express an array of inhibitory and activating receptors and the inhibitory receptors are responsible for self-tolerance while activating receptors mediate the NK cell cytotoxicity (NKCC)[21,22]. KIRs are the most important NK cell receptors, including CD94, NKG2A, CD158 and CD314, which recognize classical MHC class I [23]. In the present study, the gene expressions of CD94, NKG2A and CD158 were significantly lower than those in SAP patients and the controls, suggesting the impaired ability to protect normal cells in AMI patients. Receptors CD335 (NKp46), CD337 (NKp30), CD48 (2B4), CD314 (NKG2D) and CD319 (CRACC) are most central activating receptors and play an important role in targeting NK cell responses toward abnormal cells and eventually the cell lysis [24-27]. In our current study, gene expressions of activating receptors, CD337, CD314 and CD319 in AMI patients were significantly decreased in comparison with SAP patients and controls respectively, demonstrating that the transduction of activating signal was inhibited in patients with AMI. The cytotoxic ability of NK cells was decreased afterwards. There was no statistical difference in mRNA expression between the SAP patients and controls in inhibitory and activating receptors, indicating that the NK receptors in SAP patients was in a nearly inactive state. Previous studies found the reduced proportions of NK cells in peripheral blood of CAD, but the reason is still controversial [28-31]. The similar loss of NK cell numbers in both AMI and SAP patients were also observed in our study. Together with the notably decreased expression of NK cell biomarkers in AMI patients, different levels of reduced immunity in NK cells were demonstrated in AMI and SAP stages. In AMI patients both numbers and receptor activity were decreased, while only a deficit of quantity was found in SAP patients.

TCR is a molecule found on the surface of T lymphocytes that is responsible for recognizing antigens. The first signal for T cell activation is provided through the TCR-CD_3 [32]. In the present study, gene expressions of TCRA, TCRB, TCRG, TCRZ, CD3D, CD3E and CD3G were significantly lower in AMI group than those in SAP and control group, indicating decreased ability of TCR antigen recognition. In addition, the loss of CD_3 T cells in PBMCs was found in both AMI and SAP patients, suggesting the dysfunction of CD_3 cells in CAD, especially in AMI stage.

Naive CD_4 T cells differentiate into T helper type 1 (Th1) and T helper type 2 (Th2). Th1 cells achieve cellular immunity mainly by secreting IL2, IL12 and IFN-ã. T-bet is a Th1 transcription factor for regulating Th1 development [33]. CD195 (CCR5) and CD182 (CXCR3) are specific Th1 lymphocyte chemokine receptors [34]. Th2 cells produce IL4, IL6 and IL10 to activate B lymphocytes and generate antibodies. GATA3 is the Th2 specific transcription factor, and CCR3 together with CD294 (CRTH2) are chemokine receptors of Th2 cells [35-37]. CD366 (Tim-3) is a Th1-specific cell surface protein while CD365 (Tim-1) is Th2-specific [38,39]. The high mRNA expressions of Th1 biomarkers (IL2 and CD366) and low RNA expressions of Th2 biomarkers (IL4, IL-10, CD278 and CD294) in AMI patients suggested a shift towards Th1 dominance. The absolute increase of CD_4T cells, IL-2, IL-4, IL-6 and IFN in plasma of AMI and SAP patients showed the differential degrees of CD_4 T cell mediated cellular immunity dysfunction in AMI and SAP patients.

CD_8 T cells kill virus-infected cells and tumor cells and play a critical role in immune protection [40]. CD_8T cell is firstly activated by TCR and CD_8 binding and then co-stimulatory molecules. CD_8 T cells make the fatal attack through the perforin-granzyme, Fas-Fas ligand (FasL), and TNF-a pathways [41,42]. The presence of CD_8 T cells in atherosclerotic lesions is widely demonstrated but studies investigating their role in atherogenesis have yielded contradictory results [43,44]. In the present study, all 15 genes related to killing ability of CD_8 T cells in AMI patients were down-regulated, especially CD8A, CD8B, CD28, CD278, GZMK, GZMM, PRF1 and CASP10 were significantly down-regulated when compared with SAP and/or controls. Together with

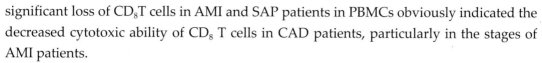

significant loss of CD₈T cells in AMI and SAP patients in PBMCs obviously indicated the decreased cytotoxic ability of CD$_8$ T cells in CAD patients, particularly in the stages of AMI patients.

We detected all 15 genes related with intracellular and extracellular markers of CD$_{19}$ B cells [45]. B cell receptor (BCR) was composed of membrane immunoglobulin (Ig) which recognizes the antigens while Igá (CD79A) and Igâ (CD79B) transmit the activation signals [46]. CD19 and CD21 are B cell co-receptors, which enhance the BCR signal transduction [47]. The B cell specific Src-family kinase CD5, specifically binding B cell surface Ig, is dispensable for B cell activation [48]. CD268 is the principal receptor required for BAFF-mediated B cell activation [49]. CD279 encodes a cell surface membrane protein of Ig superfamily and plays a role in their differentiation [50]. In AMI patients, gene expressions of CD5, CD19, CD20, CD21, CD22, CD23, CD40, CD79A, CD79B, CD268 and CD279 were significantly lower than those in SAP and/or control group, which showed that the B cell activation was blocked in AMI patients. Comparing SAP patients with the control group, there was no significant gene expression difference in B cell activation. The detection of B cell quantity, IgM and IgG levels in PBMCs were decreased in both AMI and SAP patients. In sum, in AMI patients, gene expressions and numbers of B cells were reduced, demonstrating the deeply weakened humoral immunity in AMI group.

In the present study, in AMI patients the mRNA expression of immune system was consistent with the cytological level and the decline of both parameters demonstrated the collapse of immune function in AMI group. In SAP patients, the immunity related gene expression was different from cytological level. The CH50, C3 and C4 were increased and the number of NK cells, CD$_3$, CD$_8$ T cells and CD$_{19}$ B cells was decreased, while the gene expression of immune system was in a nearly inactive status. In the current study, we can conclude that the attack of AMI and SA was associated with different levels of immune dysfunction. AMI occurs in the stage of immune collapse while SAP occurs in progressively reduced levels of immunity but still within the boundary of compensation. The quantity of immune cells in peripheral blood may reflect the current state of immune function and the gene expression of immune system stands for the compensatory capacity of immune system.

In AMI patients, the suppressed innate and adaptive immune systems, especially the cytotoxic ability, failing to remove the exogenous pathogens, was observed. Since various exogenous microorganisms' infections are supposed as risk factors of AMI [8,9] and infection seems to be linked to plaque rupture [4-7], we may conclude that the pathogenesis of AMI might be related with infections of pathogens under the depletion of immune system. That is the reason why a single vaccine is ineffective on AMI prevention. Improving the immunity of CAD patients may be considered as a potential target for medical intervention and prevention of AMI.

(published: Int J Med Sci 2017; 14(2):181-190)

References

1. Libby P, Ridker PM, Hansson GK. Progress and challenges in translating the biology of atherosclerosis. Nature. 2011; 473: 317-325.

2. Libby P, Theroux P.Pathophysiology of coronary artery disease. Circulation. 2005; 111:3481-3488.

3. Shah PK. Pathophysiology of coronary thrombosis: role of plaque rupture and plaque erosion. ProgCardiovasc Dis. 2002; 44:357-368.

4. Levi M, van der Poll T, Schultz M. New insights into pathways that determine the link between infection and thrombosis. Neth J Med. 2012; 70:114-120.

5. Chatzidimitriou D, Kirmizis D, Gavriilaki E, Chatzidimitriou M, Malisiovas N.Atherosclerosis

6. Levi M, van der Poll T, Schultz M.Infectiiion and inflammation as risk factors for thrombosis and atherosclerosis. SeminThromb Hemost. 2012; 38:506-514.

7. Khan S, Rahman HN, Okamoto T, Matsunaga T, Fujiwara Y, Sawa T, Yoshitake J, Ono K, Ahmed KA, Rahaman MM, Oyama K, Takeya M, Ida T, Kawamura Y, Fujii S, Akaike T.Promotion of atherosclerosis by Helicobacter cinaedi infection that involves macrophage-driven proinflammatory responses. Sci Rep. 2014; 4: 4680.

8. Mostafa A, Mohamed MK, Saeed M, Hasan A, Fontanet A, Godsland I, Coady E, Esmat G, El-Hoseiny M, Abdul-Hamid M, Hughes A, Chaturvedi N. Hepatitis C infection and clearance: impact on atherosclerosis and cardiometabolic risk factors. Gut. 2010; 59:1135-1140.

9. Yan WW, Zhang KS, Duan QL, Wang LM. Significantly reduced function of T cells in patients with acute arterialthrombosis. Journal of Geriatric Cardiology. 2015; 12: 287-293.

10. Yan WW, Wang LM, Jiang JF, Xu WJ, Gong Z, Duan QL, Li C, Song HM, Che L, Shen YQ, Zhou L.Differential expression of T cell-related genes in AMI and SA stages of coronary artery disease. Int J ClinExp Med. 2015; 8:10875-10884.

11. Matusik P, Guzik B, Weber C, Guzik TJ. Do we know enough about the immune pathogenesis of acute coronary syndromes to improve clinical practice? ThrombHaemost. 2012; 108:443-456.

12. Arbab-Zadeh A, Nakano M, Virmani R, Fuster V. Acute coronary events. Circulation. 2012; 125: 1147-1156.

13. Dobbin K, Simon R. Sample size determination in microarray experiments for class comparison and prognostic classification. Biostatistics. 2005; 6:27-38.

14. Thygesen K, Alpert JS, Jaffe AS, Simoons ML, Chaitman BR, White HD. Third universal definition of myocardial infarction. J Am CollCardiol. 2012; 60: 1581-1598.

15. Wiltgen M, Tilz GP.DNA microarray analysis: principles and clinical impact. Hematology. 2007; 12:271-287.

16. Cooper MA, Colonna M, Yokoyama WM. Hidden talents of natural killers: NK cells in innate and adaptive immunity. EMBO Rep. 2009; 10:1103-1110.

17. Lappegård KT, Garred P, Jonasson L, Espevik T, Aukrust P, Yndestad A, Mollnes TE, Hovland A.A vital role for complement in heart disease. Mol Immunol.2014;61:126-134.

18. Iltumur K, Karabulut A, Toprak G, Toprak N. Complement activation in acute coronary syndromes. APMIS. 2005; 113: 167-174.

19. Michael R, Cusack MB, Michael S, et al. Systemic inflammation in unstable angina is the result of myocardial necrosis. J Am CollCardiol. 2002; 39:1917-1923

20. Leinoe E, Pachai A, Brandslund I. Complement activation reaches maximum during equilibrium between antigen and antibody in an *in vitro* model for thrombolysis with streptokinase. APMIS. 2000; 10:685-688.

21. Backström E, Kristensson K, Ljunggren HG. Activation of natural killer cells: underlying molecular mechanisms revealed. Scand J Immunol. 2004; 60: 14-22.

22. Middleton D, Curran M, Maxwell L. Natural killer cells and their receptors. Transpl Immunol. 2002; 10: 147-64.

23. Campbell KS, Purdy AK. Structure/function of human killer cell immunoglobulin-like receptors: lessons from polymorphisms, evolution, crystal structures and mutations. Immunology. 2011; 132:315-325.

24. Raulet DH, Gasser S, Gowen BG, Deng W, Jung H. Regulation of ligands for the NKG2D activating receptor. Annu Rev Immunol. 2013; 31:413-441.

25. Zafirova B, Wensveen FM, Gulin M, Polić B. Regulation of immune cell function and differentiation by the NKG2D receptor. Cell Mol Life Sci. 2011; 68:3519-3529.

26. Koch J, Steinle A, Watzl C, Mandelboim O. Activating natural cytotoxicity receptors of natural killer cells in cancer and infection. Trends Immunol 2013; 34:182-191.

27. Claus M, Meinke S, Bhat R, Watzl C. Regulation of NK cell activity by 2B4, NTB-A and CRACC. Front Biosci. 2008; 13: 956-965.

28. Whitman SC, Rateri DL, Szilvassy SJ, Yokoyama W, Daugherty A. Depletion of natural killer cell function decreases atherosclerosis in low-density lipoprotein receptor null mice. Arterioscler Thromb Vasc Biol. 2004; 24:1049-1054

29. Li W, Lidebjer C, Yuan XM, Szymanowski A, Backteman K, Ernerudh J, Leanderson P, Nilsson L, Swahn E, Jonasson L. NK cell apoptosis in coronary artery disease: relation to oxidative stress. Atherosclerosis. 2008; 199:65-72.

30. Jonasson L, Backteman K, Ernerudh J. Loss of natural killer cell activity in patients with coronary artery disease. Atherosclerosis. 2005; 183:316-321.

31. Backteman K, Ernerudh J, Jonasson L. Natural killer (NK) cell deficit in coronary artery disease: no aberrations in phenotype but sustained reduction of NK cells is associated with low-grade inflammation. Clin Exp Immunol. 2014; 175:104-112.

32. Zehn D, King C, Bevan MJ, Palmer E. TCR signaling requirements for activating T cells and for generating memory. Cell Mol Life Sci. 2012; 69: 1565-1575.

33. Vanaki E, Ataei M, Sanati MH, Mansouri P, Mahmoudi M, Zarei F, JadaliZ.Expression patterns of Th1/Th2 transcription factors in patients with guttate psoriasis. Acta Microbiol Immunol Hung. 2013; 60: 163-174.

34. Gao P, Zhou XY, Yashiro-Ohtani Y, Yang YF, Sugimoto N, Ono S, Nakanishi T, Obika S, Imanishi T, Egawa T, Nagasawa T, Fujiwara H, HamaokaT. The unique target specificity of a nonpeptide chemokine receptor antagonist: selective blockade of two Th1 chemokine receptors CCR5 and CXCR3. J Leukoc Biol. 2003; 73: 273-280.

35. Wan YY. GATA3: a master of many trades in immune regulation. Trends Immunol. 2014; 35: 233-242.

36. Sallusto F, Mackay CR, Lanzavecchia A. Selective expression of the eotaxin receptor CCR3 by human T helper 2 cells. Science. 1997; 277: 2005-2007.

37. Nagata K, Hirai H. The second PGD$_2$ receptor CRTH2: structure, properties, and functions in leukocytes. Prostaglandins Leukot Essent Fatty Acids. 2003; 69: 169-177.

38. Hastings WD, Anderson DE, Kassam N, Koguchi K, Greenfield EA, Kent SC, Zheng XX, Strom TB, Hafler DA, Kuchroo VK. TIM-3 is expressed on activated human CD_4 T cells and regulates Th1 and Th17 cytokines. Eur J Immunol.2009;39:2492-2501.

39. Curtiss ML, Gorman JV, Businga TR, Traver G, Singh M, Meyerholz DK, Kline JN, Murphy AJ, Valenzuela DM, Colgan JD, Rothman PB, Cassel SL. Tim-1 regulates Th2 responses in an airway hypersensitivity model. Eur J Immunol.2012;42:651-661.

40. Gadhamsetty S, Marée AFM, Beltman JB, de Boer RJ. A General Functional Response of Cytotoxic T Lymphocyte -Mediated Killing of Target Cells. Biophys J. 2014; 106: 1780-1791.

41. Keefe D, Shi L, Feske S, Massol R, Navarro F, Kirchhausen T, Lieberman J. Perforin triggers a plasma membrane-repair response that facilitates CTL induction of apoptosis. Immunity. 2005; 23: 249-262.

42. Berke G. The CTL's kiss of death. Cell. 1995; 81: 9-12.

43. Kyaw T, Winship A, Tay C, Kanellakis P, Hosseini H, Cao A, Li P, Tipping P, Bobik A, TohBH.Cytotoxic and proinflammatory CD_8 T lymphocytes promote development of vulnerable atherosclerotic plaques in apoE-deficient mice. Circulation. 2013;127:1028-1039

44. Zhou J, Dimayuga PC, Zhao X, Yano J, Lio WM, Trinidad P, Honjo T, Cercek B, Shah PK, Chyu KY.CD8(+)CD25(+) T cells reduce atherosclerosis in apoE(−/−) mice. Biochem Biophys Res Commun. 2014;443:864-870.

45. Pike KA, Ratcliffe MJ. Cell surface immunoglobulin receptors in B cell development. Semin Immunol. 2002; 14:351-358.

46. Kurosaki T. Regulation of BCR signaling. Mol Immunol.2011; 48:1287-1291.

47. Barrington RA, Schneider TJ, Pitcher LA, Mempel TR, Ma M, Barteneva NS, Carroll MC. Uncoupling CD21 and CD19 of the B-cell coreceptor. Proc Natl Acad Sci USA. 2009; 106:14490-14495.

48. Pospisil R, Silverman GJ, Marti GE, Aruffo A, Bowen MA, Mage RG. CD5 is A potential selecting ligand for B-cell surface immunoglobulin: a possible role in maintenance and selective expansion of normal and malignant B cells. Leuk Lymphoma.2000; 36:353-365.

49. Bergmann H, Yabas M, Short A, Miosge L, Barthel N, Teh CE, Roots CM, Bull KR, Jeelall Y, Horikawa K, Whittle B, Balakishnan B, Sjollema G, Bertram EM, Mackay F, Rimmer AJ, Cornall RJ, Field MA, Andrews TD, Goodnow CC, Enders A. B cell survival, surface BCR and BAFFR expression, CD74 metabolism, and CD8-dendritic cells require the intramembraneendopeptidase SPPL2A. J Exp Med. 2013;210:31-40.

50. Thibult ML, Mamessier E, Gertner-Dardenne J, Pastor S, Just-Landi S, Xerri L, Chetaille B, Olive D. PD-1 is a novelregulator of humanB-cellactivation. Int Immunol.2013;25:129-137.

Part III
Summary and prospect

Chapter 14

Differences of origin and onset between acute venous and arterial thrombus

1. Gist of acute venous thrombosis

(1) Origin of venous thrombus results from loss of timely and effective clearance of intravenous infected cells/malignant tumor cells under the condition of systemic immune cell balancing function collapse, and infectious/non-infectious fibrinous inflammations that occurred in veins.

(2) Activated integrins β3 on platelet and β2 on white blood cell membrane adhere to their ligands such as fibrinogen to build up reversibly combined filamentous mesh structures in veins, which like intravenous biological filters act as a compensatory physical defense for the human body. The function of these filters is to prevent intravenous infected cells/malignant tumor cells from going back to the whole circulation system. Red thrombi form when blood cells, mainly red blood cells, flow back and fulfill filters. Venous thrombi can cause pulmonary thromboembolism when they go into pulmonary arteries.

(3) Reversible filamentous mesh structures form under a sluggish blood flow, which are hard to be established with a quick blood flow. Integrin β2 on white blood cell membrane combines with its ligand X, which is transformed into Xa to promote fibrinogen into fibrins and thus make the biological filters firm.

(4) Mechanisms of acquired and familial venous thromboembolism are the same.

(5) Infected cells/malignant cells in veins can be cleared timely and effectively in people with sound immune cell balancing functions, and therefore there is no need to build up a physical defense like biological filters, thus venous thrombotic events will not happen.

2. Gist of acute arterial thrombosis

Comparison of genome results between arterial thrombus group and control group indicates integrated and directional changes of imunne cell blancing function collapse in acute arterial thrombotic diseases.

Research results of human genome presented a set of significantly differently expressed genes. Expression of T cell related genes is down-regulated significantly; TCR genes related with recognition and combination with antigen were down-regulated significantly; genes related with activities of MHC Ⅱ receptors were down-regulated significantly; cell killing ability of CTL was decreased; genes related to TH1/Th2/Th7/Treg were expressed significantly differently; responses of Th1 were up-regulated; Th2, Th17 and Treg immune responses were significantly down-regulated; expression of Nk cell related genes was down-regulated significantly; expression of complement genes related with caspase responses was interrupted; expression of B cell related genes lost balance significantly; expression of chemotaxis and adhesion functions of neutrophils and monocytes related genes were up-regulated significantly, indicating that acute arterial thrombotic events may be infectious responses occurring under a situation of systemic immune cell balancing function collapse.

Systemic immune cell balancing function collapse is that immune cells lose functions or immune cell balancing functions significantly decrease. Systemic immune cell balancing function collapse in patients with acute arterial thrombi indicates that the immune system cannot eliminate pathogenic microorganism or malignant cells effectively and timely. However, objectives with malignancies were excluded in this study. Logistic thinking of the author judged that it could only be explained by that stayed bacterial-like pathogenic microorganisms have not been eliminated timely and effectively in artery. Therefore, acute arterial thrombotic events may be results of accidental injury caused by active oxygen from neutrophils. Decreased activities of MHC Ⅱ receptors indicate decreased abilities of presenting bacterial antigen information. Basic law of inflammatory responses caused by bacterial microorganisms is chemotaxis and aggregation of neutrophils, and transformation from rolling adhesion to stationarity adhesion of arterial endothelial cells. The life time of neutrophils is 1-3 days, rupture of which could release plentiful active oxygen, causing undifferentiated damages to surrounding tissues, including damages to arterial intima cells, at the same time of killing bacteria. Arteries are battlefields of neutrophils and pathogens, and active oxygen might be the culprit causing arterial intima injuries. After inflammatory injuries to intima (damages and rupture of soft plaque caps, and superficial erosion), platelets adhere and aggregate to injured parts, and are involved in repair of arterial intima, which is also a process of thrombus formation. Pathogens can be cleared timely and effectively in people with sound immune cell balancing functions. As a results, arterial thrombotic events usually do not take place in such people.

The decrease of immune cell function is consistent with the genome down-regulation in AMI patients with significant decrease of the immune cell function. In SAP patients, immune cell function is decreased but genome expression is stable.

Acute aterial thrombosis and stable angina pectoris may be the products of different immune function status. AMI results from collaposed immune cell balance function, while stable angina pectoris results from gradually decreasing function of immune cells, although it is still under relative stable condition of immune cell balance. Clinical immune cell count suggests the status of immune cell function, while systemic genomic mRNA expression suggests potential compensatory ability of immune cells.

3. Similarities and differences of internal and external factors between acute venous and arterial thrombosis

General and systemic immune cell results of these studies showed that common characteristics of acute venous and arterial thrombosis are intravascular inflammatory responses under a condition of systemic immune cell balancing collapse. Venous thrombosis is intravenous infectious inflammation (virus, bacteria and so on)/ non-infectious fibrinous inflammation (malignant tumor) process, while arterial thrombosis may be extracellular pathogen infectious inflammatory process in arterial wall. Neutrophils and platelets play important roles in initiating venous and arterial thrombosis.

The origin and onset of acute venous thrombi are that intravenous infected cells and malignant cells cannot be effectively cleared, mainly shown as function lose of immune cells balancing. The formation of intravenous biological filters is a fibrinous inflammatory process to intercept pathological cells to prevent them from flowing back to the whole body. The origin and onset of acute arterial thrombi may be extracellular pathogens that cannot be effectively cleared. Arteries become battlefield of pathogens and phagocytes. Neutrophils sacrifice and release active oxygen to kill pathogens as well as arterial intima cells, and thus platelets adhere and aggregate at injured arterial endothelial cells. Formation of thrombus, no matter venous or arterial thrombosis, is an imbalance of substitution process of physical defensive function, which is shown as a thrombus disease.

Under a situation of systemic immune cell balancing function collapse, there is a high possibility of having thrombotic diseases. However, it is hard to predict when it may occur, and whether it is venous or arterial thrombus will depend on the species, quantity, virulence of the pathogens or the intravenous invasive malignant cells. Clearing pathogenic microorganisms or malignant cells by human force makes us running after diseases, while to maintain dynamic immune cell balancing function is the true essence of preventing thrombotic diseases.

Chapter 15

Epilogue: To make it simple

Are chronic diseases the choice of nature, consequence of human behavior or consequence of human living together with nature, during the process of human evolution? Undoubtedly, this is the dynamic equilibrium of lives, including human beings and their living environment.

The clinical disease spectrum has changed a lot so far and the average life span of the human being is increasing. On the other hand, the number of people with chronic diseases is still increasing, especially after a booming social economy and an elevated living standard brought about by global industrialization. However, without knowing the overall perspective of a disease, we could be always running after diseases.

Why are people sick, is it due to self-defects or choices of nature? Shown as self-defects, congenital defect (excluding human factors) is a choice of nature actually, which is an evolution form hard to be accepted. There are many kinds of human diseases, most of which are with unknown etiologies and mechanisms. Thus, evidence based medicine is the way to approach the nature of diseases. It is to avoid diseases to raise risk factor and risk stratification of diseases, which is used in modern medicine usually. Treating symptoms is the choice at present, and dot thinking and linear thinking become normalcy.

Why aren't people sick? There is a blockage wall between health and diseases. Evolution has given people this anti-disease wall, but could we recognize and understand the wall inside human bodies? The true face of a mountain is lost to my sight, for it is right in this mountain that I reside. Skin and mucosa are the defending organs, and the normal flora balances the health status. Immune defense is to exempt diseases: people are born with inner immunity, while adaptive immunity is acquired after birth. The truth is that the anti-disease wall generated along human evolution is the inner fortress of avoiding diseases, the existence of which is a cornerstone of health. To maintain the inner fortress is to keep healthy.

Thrombotic diseases belong to categories of chronic diseases. Thrombotic diseases are caused by subversive collapse of systemic immune cell function, such as collapse of inner fortress. Whether there are thrombotic diseases or not, whether they defer or not, and what is degree of cure, depend on conditions of the inner fortress or degree of its reconstruction. In another word, they all depend on conditions of immune cell functions and their degree of recovery. Immune cell balancing function differs from each other, as well as the reserve capacity of the function determines strength of individuals preventing diseases. And this is a choice of nature. When mentality and behavior of human surpass the choice continuously, nerve-endocrine-immune system regulation loses balance. Thus, subversive collapse of immune defense occurs, and then subversive diseases come, including thrombotic diseases. Though there are various kinds of diseases, the principle comes to one point. This principle indicates that a chronic disease is the results of mentality and behavior imbalance, and chronic diseases could be prevented, and health is a harmonious stage of human's internal status, society and nature.

Aging becomes a truth nowadays, while the predicted future trend is more severe. Aging brings degeneration of body structures and functions, and the same with immune organs, immune tissues, and immune cells. Essence of immune cell balancing function degeneration is consuming immune function reserve, which is irresistible and determines scales of lives. However, it is possible to control the scale finitely by avoiding overstress in body and mind, keeping optimistic mind, eating balanced food, exercising according to oneself. It is the choice of humans to postpone degeneration of human tissues and functions, and degeneration of immune cell function reserve. Young people with venous and arterial thrombus are related to excessive stress closely. Overdraft of mentality and stamina is actually overdraft of systemic function reserve, including immune system function reserve. When the anti-disease wall inside human body collapses, diseases will happen. A Chinese ancient medical rishis said, "internal health keeps diseases far away", which indicates a principle of "to make every simple".